HOW TO ACE THE
PHYSICIAN ASSISTANT
SCHOOL INTERVIEW

HOW TO ACE THE
PHYSICIAN ASSISTANT
SCHOOL INTERVIEW

Second Edition

From the author of the best-selling book
*The Ultimate Guide to Getting Into
Physician Assistant School*

Andrew J. Rodican, PA-C

Founder, AJR Associates, LLC
Northford, CT 06472
andrewrodican.com

This book is dedicated to the memory of my father,
James A. Rodican

I also dedicate this book to my wife, my children,
my daughter-in-law, my granddaughter, my siblings,
and my best friends.

As I type these words, I am on medical leave
for a significant surgery I had two short months ago.
The love and support of my family and friends
has been overwhelming.

Contents

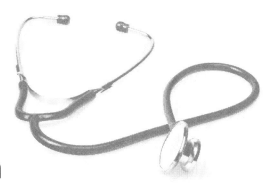

Introduction

Congratulations! You've made it to the interview phase of the PA school application process and your chances of getting accepted have increased dramatically. A typical PA program receives a thousand or more applications for a precious twenty-five-to fifty slots each cycle. Your chance of acceptance at this point is roughly two-and-one-half to five percent for any given program. Many programs invite approximately two hundred applicants to interview. If you're invited, your chances have now increased to twelve-and one-half to twenty-five percent; much better odds. Your job now is to claim your seat in the upcoming class by being the most prepared applicant in the room that day. You've taken control of your situation, and rather than be one of the thousand faceless drones trying to break into the PA profession, you've decided to do more—*be* more! At last, you're not just making positive steps in the way you interview, you're making positive steps toward getting accepted to PA school and entering your chosen profession!

So, go ahead and pat yourself on the back; you've worked hard to get here, and you deserve to be very proud of yourself. This is just the beginning, however, not the end. You now must take all the knowledge and expertise I will provide you and reduce it into a condensed, manageable format within the framework of the questions that you will be asked. You may feel a bit anxious and overwhelmed at this point, but trust me, I'm going to break all the knowledge I present in each chapter into easy-to-digest, bite-sized nuggets of valuable information that will make you the perfect PA school applicant.

Coming into the home stretch, I'll show you how to really supercharge your entire interview using targeted answers to questions you will encounter during your PA school interview. You will discover how using the PA program's various web properties (Program Website, Facebook, Google, Blogs, etc.) to uncover the Qualities and Multipliers (more on this later) that will set you apart from everyone else. This is the most important part of my tailoring method, and ultimately the technique that has helped me coach thousands of PA school applicants to success.

I'm going to teach you how to infuse these Qualities into your answers in order to tailor your responses to the program which you are interviewing with. In this book, I will take you to another level. A level that only Perfect Applicants can reach.

I want you to think of the PA school interview process like studying for a test in school. To pass the test, you need to study the material. Imagine knowing the questions on that test before taking it? Well, I'm going to provide you with the questions *and* answers. And not just carbon copy answers. I'm going to show you how to tailor your answers relative to the specific PA program that you are interviewing with. This book is the secret weapon you need to blow away the competition and get accepted into the PA school of your choice.

I've compiled the most commonly asked questions that you may be asked, along with examples of Qualities and Multipliers that you can use to improve your responses. *The answers to the questions I provide are only examples, not to be memorized verbatim. You will need to do the work and dig deep to find the Qualities and Multipliers for each program you interview with to determine what they value most.* Additionally, the answers I supply are just suggestions. They have my proven methodology behind them, making each a solid answer that the admissions committee would want to hear, but they're not necessarily one hundred percent the right answers for you. This is a guide; use it to mold your own answers based on your firsthand experiences, qualities, and values. Don't memorize the answers in this chapter; you will come off as fake and unnatural during your interview. Use this book as a springboard to help you rise above the competition and make a favorable impression on the admissions committee.

In addition to giving samples of the most common questions and answers, I'm also including the most common DOs and DON'Ts for each question, which will provide some additional insight and make answering the question much easier.

Remember: *Tailoring the interview to the program you are interviewing with is the most important thing.*

In the first chapter of this second edition of *How to Ace the Physician Assistant School Interview*, I'm going to teach you the "Tailoring Method," a powerful technique that provides the framework for any interview question and will help you go from a vanilla applicant to the Perfect Applicant!

In the second section of the book, I'll cover several interview questions, including:

- ► Traditional Questions
- ► Behavioral Questions
- ► Situational Questions
- ► Ethical Questions
- ► Illegal Questions

This section is basically an up-to-date, how-to on interviewing for PA school. Of course, before you even walk into that interview, there are some key steps that you should take to make sure you're presenting the whole package and getting off on the right foot...and I'll help you nail those, too!

The third section is solely dedicated to the Multiple Mini Interview (MMI), described by many applicants as the most difficult type of interview. There are an infinite number of possible MMI questions, tasks, and role-playing scenarios, so it is imperative that you learn a blueprint for answering any of them. I provide you with an exact blueprint in this chapter.

The final chapters deal with information beyond answering interview questions, but are possibly more important. You will learn the secret to making yourself likeable at your interview.

In chapter 8, Winning through High Impact Communication, I'm going to teach you the secret to achieving a top score on your interview. If you don't fully understand this secret before you enter the interview room, you can answer all the questions correctly, but still not achieve a high score. This chapter will teach the components of the verbal, vocal, and visual parts of the interview, including which component is most important.

In the next chapter, *Before the Interview*, I'm going to give you some tips on preparing for the interview right up until you walk into the building. I'll also include how to deal with anxiety and what you should do the night before.

I'll then cover *Dressing for Interviews*. This chapter will take away the guesswork while deciding what to wear to your interview. As a seven-year military veteran, I was always a stickler for the dress code. I looked an applicant over from hair, to suit, to nails, and to shoes. After reading this chapter, you'll know exactly how to make a favorable first impression.

Finally, I'm going to cover twenty of the most commonly asked questions by PA school applicants concerning the interview process. These questions and answers are laid out for you, so you don't have to go searching multiple other sources for them.

NOTE: It is a smart idea to find out if your interview is going to be "open" or "closed." In other words, an *open* interview means the committee members will have access to your CASPA application. A *closed* interview means that the interviewers will not have access to your CASPA file.

In a closed interview, you will, especially, want to be sure and highlight some of the key accomplishments or information that you want the committee members to know about you.

To find out if your interview is open or closed, you can call the PA program office, or send an email.

I wish you all the best of luck on your journey to become a PA, and I hope we will meet one day as colleagues.

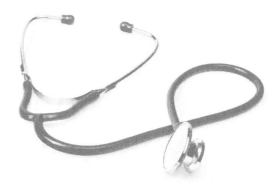

CHAPTER 1

The Tailoring Method

In this chapter, I'll introduce you to a powerful tool that will help you leave the competition in the dust: The Tailoring Method. I will also explain the idea of the Perfect Applicant. More importantly, I'll introduce the most important pieces to the "interview question puzzle," the Qualities and Multipliers.

If you've read any of my books, you've probably noticed that I do things a little differently than anyone else. As the pioneer in PA school applicant coaching and author of the first book to hit the market in 1996, *The Ultimate Guide to Getting Into Physician Assistant School,* I use specialized techniques and training to help applicants get accepted. There are many more PA school *coaches* available now than when I started; however, none have the longevity, experience, and knowledge that I've gained over the past twenty years working with applicants from all over the country. Yes, I help applicants get accepted!

Okay, so what is my secret? How have I been able to teach so many applicants to succeed, where others have failed on their own in the past? Because there is one key to success that I teach those I coach:

It's not about you, it's about *them*!

You may think it's about you. After all, you really have a strong passion to become a physician assistant. You've completed all the prerequisites for PA school, you have a 3.7 science GPA, 3000 hours of hands-on medical experience, phenomenal GRE scores, and excellent references. You're ready to prove that you have what it takes during the interview.

But it's not about *you*; It's about meeting the needs of the program(s) where you apply and demonstrating that you have exactly what they are looking for in a Perfect Applicant. The interviewer(s) look to see if you have the qualities to become a great student and a great PA. More importantly, they want to be certain you will be a good classmate, complete the rigorous program, pass your boards, and be a respected representative of their program out in the community.

Many other PAs, friends, coworkers, and PA school coaches will tell you that the best thing you can do at your interview is summarize your past experiences and highlight your personal strengths and accomplishments. And, to be honest, when those strengths and experiences are better than the other applicants, it's often enough to get accepted.

This is not my philosophy. This is the "old school" way of interviewing. What if you don't have a clear-cut advantage over the other applicants? In the huge applicant pool, there will be the best of the best at the interview, and *everyone* will have a strong resume.

What if you sit across from the interviewer and go on and on about your accomplishments, thinking you are the perfect applicant, not knowing that what you're saying is irrelevant to what the interviewer and the program is looking for?

The program already knows exactly the type of applicant they're going to accept long before you enter the interview room. Many of the interviewers have been doing this for a long time. They instinctively know the qualities and traits the program desires. They obviously don't know the specific name of the applicants they are going to accept but take my word for it: They know the type of person they want, and more importantly, they know the strengths and qualities that this person *must* possess.

The question is: How do you become that person the program likes to accept? How do you demonstrate the qualities that the program values most? How do you make the admissions committee's (ADCOMs) job easy?

You must point out ways you can be of value to the program, namely, how you can help them achieve their goals based upon your past training and experience. You'll get your reward if they invite you to join the upcoming class. But, you must be more interested in them than you are in yourself. Be there for them. Take it from my own experience being on an admissions committee, it's a tough job. The perfect applicants make the interviewers' job easy, but so do the vanilla applicants.

But how does one do this?

By using my Tailoring Method, of course!

At this point it should be clear that the program you are about to interview with already knows the type of person they want to accept into their upcoming class. I like to refer to this person as their *Perfect Applicant*.

The Perfect Applicant

You are going to see this term a lot throughout the book, and that is because my goal is to transform you into this person before you set foot into the interview room.

What is the Perfect Applicant? As I've already said, every PA program has a certain type of person in mind when it comes to the applicants they will accept. The person will need to have several specific *Qualities* that the program values or puts a lot of emphasis on. When the program is conducting interviews, they will normally select the person who best exemplifies those Qualities, specific qualities they are looking for. This person is their Perfect Applicant.

I use a fun mathematical equation to show what makes up a PA:

$$PA = (A + Q)^m$$

I know that you're probably thinking, "Please, I completed all of my prerequisites! No more math!" Don't worry, this is the only equation you'll have to remember, and I promise there will be no numbers involved.

More than anything it's just a fun way to represent what makes up the Perfect Applicant. It will make more sense after we break down the components.

A = Answer

Simply stated, the A in the equation refers to your answer to the question that the interviewer asks. In a lot of cases, this will be a success story from your past, one that clearly demonstrates an example of you succeeding in your past jobs or any relevant scenarios.

And while I'm discussing success stories, remember this: It's always a good idea to go into every interview armed with a few of these up your sleeve. Everybody experiences a moment when his or her mind draws a blank during an interview. For these instances, it helps to have a few pre-selected success stories to fall back on. At the very least, you can spin an uncomfortable silence into a positive by telling a story that demonstrates a success you've had in the past.

Q = Qualities

Qualities are what make up the Perfect Applicant. These are generally different types of knowledge, skills, or abilities that the program considers to be of utmost importance. These are the things that you must reference or exemplify in the interview to set yourself apart from the competition.

As I mentioned earlier, an interviewer will have a set of Qualities in mind that their Perfect Applicant must have. It is your job to find out what these Qualities are, and then demonstrate to the admissions committee that you possess them. I'll show you how to find these in the next section of this chapter. I'll also show you how to infuse Qualities into your answers for various interview questions.

Here is a brief list of Qualities that PA programs look for in a strong candidate:

- Teamwork
- Empathy
- Ability to handle stress
- Community service
- Working with the underserved
- Passion for becoming a PA
- Motivation to become a PA
- Diversity
- Judgment
- Emotional stability

- Adaptability
- Compassion
- Maturity
- Detail oriented
- Interpersonal skills
- Communication skills
- Autonomy
- Hard worker
- Effective listener
- Life-long learner
- Healthcare experience

m = Multipliers

Multipliers act as bonus points in your interview; they will boost your answers from good to great! Multipliers are tidbits of information that the interviewer is not expecting you to know. This would include things like special programs, initiatives, or events, to name a few. The *m* acts as an exponent, because it increases your chance of being the Perfect Applicant exponentially!

The reason these are so effective is that they help you demonstrate your level of knowledge of the program and its culture, and really make a statement about the amount of preparation you've done. To take it a step further, Multipliers can make you look like you are already a student in the eyes of the interviewer.

I'll show you exactly how to find Multipliers in the next section.

Does that make sense? Let's just go over the general idea for those of us who feel like passing out whenever they see an equation. So now we have:

$$\text{Perfect Applicant} = (\text{Answer} + \text{Quality})^{\text{multiplier}}$$

When an admissions committee member asks you a question in the interview, they will be expecting you to respond. You have a choice. You can either give them a straight, literal answer that is your best attempt at giving them the information they need. *Or,* you can utilize my Tailoring Method, and answer the question by infusing your response with a Quality (A + Q) that you know the program is looking for in their Perfect Applicant, and *then* put the icing on the cake by including a multiplier (m)!

The truth of the matter is, your competition won't stand a chance if they are just using the "old school" interview techniques.

So, obviously, the next logical question is: How do you find out the specific Qualities that a program is looking for?

This is the key. You simply can't guess which qualities you think the program *might* put a lot of value in. You must know exactly. If you try to be clever and emphasize a Quality that your program doesn't care about, you're just going to sound like—well, let's just say that it's not going to help your cause.

In the next section, I'll show you how I identify which Qualities your program values. At the same time, it will reveal how to find some of the multipliers that you need to demonstrate your knowledge!

Finding Qualities and Multipliers

Now that we are all in agreement that it is essential to respond to interview questions by infusing the program's desired Perfect Applicant Qualities into our answers, the next step is to figure out what these Qualities and Multipliers are, *and* where they can be found.

As you can probably imagine, PA school interview preparation has evolved greatly alongside the proliferation of technology; namely, the Internet and social media. When I applied to PA school, the only way I could get information on the programs I was applying to was in the literature they provided, by attending the open house, or calling with questions—I know, I'm really dating myself! Similarly, doing program research was pretty much limited to brochures, the printed *PA Programs Directory,* and by asking PAs in the workforce. Not exactly "top secret" information! Almost everyone walked into an interview on an even playing field, because there simply wasn't the infrastructure for sharing information like there is today.

Luckily for you, times have changed. Information is more easily accessible than at any other time in the past fifty years of the PA profession. The exponential growth of the Internet has not only paved the way for exponential growth in the amount of information at our fingertips, but also revolutionized the connectivity between PA programs and their prospective students.

Black-and-white brochures have been replaced with websites. Using photos, videos, and other interesting multimedia, organizations are now able to give prospective students a glimpse into their culture, so that even before one walks into the interview room, he or she already has a good idea of what it will be like to attend the program.

But that's not all.

They also leave clues. What kind of clues? The kind of clues that are *very* interesting to me, and from now on, will be very interesting to you. This is where we begin to dig around for potential Qualities and Multipliers, the life-blood of my Tailoring Method and perhaps the most influential part of a successful PA school interview, beginning with a PA program's website.

Now, I can imagine you might be thinking, "Really Andy? Look for information on a program's website? Not exactly a revolutionary idea..." You'd be surprised how many of my coaching applicants thought the same thing at the beginning.

But it's not just about gathering some background information on your PA program of choice, or simply studying their mission statement before heading into your interview. When I say that they are leaving clues on their website, I mean it. One of the absolute best places to discover the types of Qualities that their Perfect Candidate must possess is on their website, and this is how you do it.

General Information

Begin by navigating the website of the PA program you are interviewing with. Once you reach the home page, it's important that you get a good feel for all the general information that is available, including:

- Mission of the program
- Vision of the program
- About Us
- Prerequisites
- PANCE pass/fail rates
- Admissions
- Curriculum
- Accreditation
- Is there a cadaver lab?
- Is it affiliated with a medical school?

Now to recap, these are just the basics. Nothing about learning this information will set you apart from your competitors, but you'll sure set yourself apart (the wrong way) if you don't know this stuff inside and out. You need to get a general feel for what the program includes, what they value, and any relevant current events or news stories that they may be mentioned in.

Having said that, take notice of any themes that jump out at you. I have found that occasionally, Qualities and Multipliers can be found among the general information, depending on how the program chooses to present themselves to the public. For example, you may get a sense that "giving back to the community" is important to a school based on headlines or articles found on a program's home page. Take note of anything that the program is going out of their way to share.

Finding Qualities

Once you feel you have a solid understanding of the general information, the next thing you need to do is drill down to get more interview-focused information. This is where the "About Us" page usually comes into play.

Most programs have a link, usually located on the home page, that will take you directly to everything program-related. It can usually be found under such headings as "About the PA Program," "Curriculum," and other links like "Research" or "Student Life."

Why are these pages so great for finding Qualities and Multipliers? Well, because it is there that programs really begin the process of sharing their mission, values, and beliefs for what makes their Perfect Applicant. Why do they do this? The main reason is to attract the right kind of applicants. At Duke, they want to show the Qualities that make up a "Duke PA program student" with hopes that they will attract similar candidates (and weed out those who aren't up to par).

Similarly, a program works very hard to establish and identify their "culture" (the beliefs and behaviors that determine how a program's students and faculty interact, usually reflected in things such as community service, faculty credentials, and curriculum), and the "About Our Program" page is an excellent medium to achieve this.

What does this mean for you, the interviewee? This is a *crucial* step. As I've mentioned earlier in this book, you absolutely need to tailor your responses to the program you are interviewing with, and you do this by infusing Qualities and Multipliers into your answers. Some of these very important elements can easily be found on the Home Page or "About Our Program" page.

On page 10, the sidebar *What We Look for In an Applicant* illustrates what Qualities were mentioned on the Duke PA program Admissions page. You will notice in the description that the program has hinted (even more than hinted, almost shouted) how important it is for them to find **diversity**, **community service**, and **students from underserved areas**. You will also notice many other Qualities that Duke values in the Perfect Applicant.

How would your qualifications match Duke's profile?

Duke's PA program values **community service**; therefore, it's important that you can *demonstrate* that you possess this Quality.

How do you do this?

What We Look for In an Applicant

As the population of the United States becomes increasingly diverse, cultural diversity within the PA profession is critical. The PA Program is committed to recruiting and matriculating a wide range of students including but not limited to those who are underrepresented in the PA profession because PAs interact with patients, families and communities from diverse backgrounds. We strive to create an educational environment conducive to collaborative learning through shared experiences and skills from each member of the class. The heterogeneity of the class provides a powerful platform for introducing students to the complex and diverse nature of health care. Applicants are reviewed holistically for their unique experiences, leadership potential and commitment to education.

The Duke PA program is a mission driven program that recruits caring individuals who provide competent health care. We value applicants who demonstrate a heart for service and a commitment to increasing access to health care. We give preference to applicants who demonstrate a strong match to our mission.

Applicants who have served their communities or their countries through volunteer activities, military service, employment opportunities or service oriented programs greatly enhance the cultural perspective of the class. The PA Program is committed to attracting students from geographically underserved regions such as Area Health Education Centers (AHEC) in North Carolina, as well as students from different racial, ethnic, and socioeconomic backgrounds. The PA Program also values diversity in other forms such as age, gender, gender identity, disability and years of experience in the health care field.

QUALITIES NOTED

Cultural Diversity

Students underrepresented in the PA profession

Collaboration

Leadership

Commitment to education

Heart for service

Strong match for our vision

Service oriented

Students from geographically underserved regions in North Carolina

Students from different racial, ethnic, and socioeconomic backgrounds

Years of health care experience

Source: "What We Look for in an Applicant." Department of Community and Family Medicine in the Duke University School of Medicine, cfm.duke.edu/duke-physician-assistant-program/admissions/what-we-look-applicant

By carefully infusing one of your answers with this quality. For example, see the tailored answer to the response below based on the Quality identified in the sidebar:

Q: You've been accepted to another program already. Why haven't you accepted their offer?

A: I feel very fortunate to be accepted to XYZ PA program, but I want to find a program like this one where I will truly be able to add value. I've been focused on a program that is a leader in the area I'm most passionate about: community service.

Now, keep this in mind: A program can reveal their desired Perfect Applicant Qualities in many ways. You can find Qualities in YouTube videos, Facebook, Google, articles, and student blog posts. You can find them on one of the many tabs on the Home Page. The point is, you really must dig around to see what you can turn up. Trust me, it's in your best interest!

In the Question and Answer portion of this book, I'll show you many examples of how to tailor your responses to the program where you are interviewing, by using Qualities.

Multipliers

The way you find Multipliers on a program's website is not like searching for Qualities. The "About Us" page is certainly a wonderful place to get started, but while the Qualities the program desires in the Perfect Candidate seem to jump off the page at you (a lot of these programs like to boast, after all...) the Multipliers are not something that will necessarily be as obvious. Why? Well, mainly because they don't even know that Multipliers exist. Rather, they don't expect you, the interviewee, to zone in on them and like a ninja, use them as a secret weapon in your interview.

As I've said before, Multipliers are like the "cherry on top" of your interview answer. This is where you really get to flex your muscles and show the interviewer *you* have a deeper understanding of the program than the other applicants. Therefore, it's important for you to focus on things like the program's upcoming (or past) events, special programs that they offer or any outreach programs or initiatives that they support.

Here are two excerpts of possible Multipliers (highlighted in bold) taken from a Google search on Duke's PA program. You won't find these multipliers on Duke's website:

PA Students Aid Underserved Communities

Each year, Duke's Physician Assistant Program awards eight second-year students the Underserved Community Scholarship (UCS). As part of and HRSA-funded grant project, the scholarship requires students to complete their clinical rotations in an underserved community of North Carolina.

In today's post, Faviola Rubio-Cespedes guest blogs about her experience as a Duke fellow at CommWell Health in Dunn, NC:

From a young age, I knew that I wanted to pursue a career in medicine. However, for a long time, I didn't know how to make that dream a reality. After graduating from college, my desire to help others led me to join the Peace Corps. I was stationed in Guatemala where I served as a rural health volunteer at a local clinic. During this time, I noticed physician assistants performing physical examinations, ordering diagnostic studies, and analyzing and managing treatments for patients. I quickly became interested in the profession, and ultimately enrolled in the Duke PA program in 2011.

In February, I was accepted as an Underserved Community Scholar and assigned to complete my rotations at ComWell Health in Dunn County. At the clinic, my key role is to take histories, examine patients, present patients to my preceptor, recommend treatment options and develop SOAP notes. However, the opportunities are endless. In addition to my core responsibilities, I've had the opportunity to deliver babies, aid with cervical biopsies, first-assist with C-sections, perform incision and drainage of abscesses, etc.

Similar to the Peace Corps, this scholarship program has enabled me to impact health care on a community level. It has also given me a deeper understanding of the effects of population constraints like low health literacy, poverty, homelessness and lack of insurance. By observing the providers at ComWell Health, I've learned how to get necessary tests and medications for patients with financial difficulties. I've also learned to maximize every appointment because there's no guarantee that a patient will return, especially in Dunn, where there is a high volume of migrant workers

I highly recommend that my peers apply to the Duke PA program, especially if they have a history with Americorps or Peace Corps and/or are seeking to impact a community.

Source: Duke PA Program blogger, 7/25/13.

Bringing up one of these things in your response, especially **Duke's Underserved Community Scholarship**, really shows that you have done your research, but also gives the interviewer the feeling that you are already "one of them." You bridge the gap between being a candidate and a student by showing your level of comfort and understanding with the way the organization does things. Using the same question as above, see the new answer with the multiplier in bold.

Q: You've been accepted to another program already. Why haven't you accepted their offer?

A: I feel very fortunate to be accepted to XYZ PA program, but I want to find a program like this one where I will truly be able to add value. I've been focused on a program that is a leader in the area I'm most passionate about: community service and working with underserved populations. **In fact, what drew my attention initially was an article and student bog post I read, concerning the fact that Duke's PA program admits eight**

second-year students to its Underserved Community Scholarship (USC) Program. These students spend their clinical rotations in underserved communities, and I feel that my values are shared by those belonging to Duke's PA program.

How many other applicants do you think will have read this post before their interview?

Final Thought on Qualities and Multipliers

At the end of the day, finding Qualities and Multipliers on a program's website (and specifically, their "About our Program" page) is not especially difficult. And, if you take the time to really explore the program's website, the program's Facebook page, student blogs, Google, and even YouTube videos—making sure to leave no stone unturned—you will be sure to find the Qualities and Multipliers you need to position yourself as the Perfect Applicant.

Here's the thing: Most applicants stop at the program's website (if they even do that). The program's website is not the only place that you'll find Qualities and Multipliers relative to the program. As you can imagine, the Internet is a vast resource and there is a lot of information. Use all the media I mention in the previous paragraph to find Qualities and Multipliers, and you will be way ahead of the competition!

Another perfect way to find Qualities and Multipliers relative to the program, is to attend the Open House, and ask faculty and students directly what Qualities the program values most. If you can also learn about some Multipliers, all the better.

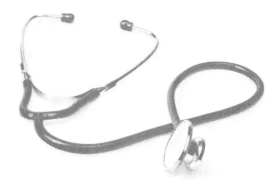

CHAPTER 2

Traditional Questions

Now that we've covered my Tailoring Method and how to infuse Qualities and Multipliers into your interview answers, it's time to get to the part of the book you've been waiting for: The questions and answers you're going to face when you're sitting in the hot seat.

Before we discuss the questions themselves, let's talk about two distinct types of questions the admissions committees will ask you. Questions usually fall into one of two categories: traditional interview questions and behavioral—or competency—interview questions. Traditional interview questions also include situational interview questions, ethical interview questions, and illegal interview questions. If you're a reapplicant, or you've had an interview for a job at all in the past few years, you'll recognize some of the questions covered in this chapter.

Traditional interview questions attempt to find out the kind of person you are while also exploring your professional attitudes, aptitudes, and qualifications. These are usually simple questions like *Why did you apply to our program?*, *Why do you want to become a PA?*, or *How do you stay current on the PA profession?*

Behavioral questions, on the other hand, are trickier. These kinds of questions are based on psychology, which states that the way you behaved in the past is an accurate predictor of the way you are going to behave in the future. Statistically, that is true. For instance, when police are trying to sniff out a suspect, someone with a history of criminal activity can become a prime suspect. Once someone is shown to have broken the law, it is statistically likely that he or she will do it again at some point.

You are a "prime suspect" for acceptance into the interviewer's school, and by asking about how you've responded to situations in the past, the interviewer can help predict how successfully you will respond to similar situations that may occur as a PA student in their program.

Behavioral questions can really catch you off guard if you aren't used to them and haven't prepared for them. They require a lot more thinking than traditional interview questions. "How do you handle stress?" (a traditional-type question) is a lot easier to answer than "Describe a time when you had to handle a stressful situation" (a behavioral-type question).

Behavioral questions are more probing than traditional interview questions; they seem to be inviting you to open up and be more of a human personality to the interviewer.

Behavioral questions may even seem like trick questions, because they require you to do some thinking, and might even require some soul-searching—something you don't want to be doing in front of the interviewer while she silently times you and realizes you don't know what the heck you're talking about. You really need to be prepared beforehand for behavioral-type questions. Winging them is simply not an option—you may find yourself falling face-first into the turf.

You can easily be tripped up by the unexpected quality of behavioral-type questions. You may not be able to think of anything and will look (and feel) like a fish out of water, with its mouth gaping, if you are not prepared. Thinking on your feet in an interview setting, while it's sometimes necessary, is far too risky.

Look at politicians and other public figures like celebrities. Because so much depends on their image, almost everything they say is carefully scripted. They prepare and practice everything from the words they will use, to the inflection they put in their voice, to the expression they will have on their faces, even down to the gestures they make with their hands. They prepare "statements"; they rarely speak entirely off the cuff. You must be prepared on all these fronts as well (without seeming unnatural about it), or else you may blurt something out that makes you look bad or say one thing with your mouth and quite another with your facial expressions or body language. (I will cover this extensively in Chapter 8, Winning Through High-Impact Communication.)

Chatting happily on, flattered by the interviewer's interest, you may give too much information: "It's interesting you asked me about a time I encountered a stressful situation and how I handled it. Now that I think about it, I was considering taking a class in stress reduction techniques after I had to take a sabbatical at my last job because of being too stressed out."

Uh-oh.

That's why I wrote this book—not to make you into a phony, but to give you a heads-up on the kinds of questions you may encounter during interviews, both behavioral and traditional, to help you craft some model answers, and get you thinking about how you can tailor your responses using your own experiences into winning frameworks.

I'll also provide you with some big "No-Nos" to look out for. I'll give you some outlines of structures into which you can fit your specific information and come off like a song, no matter what kind of question is thrown at you. I'll provide clues as to what the interviewer is really getting at with his or her question and how to successfully navigate the dimly lit waters. I'll also give you hints and guidance on what *not* to say.

Remember the general principle to apply to any interviewing situation: "It's not about you, it's about *them*." If you don't learn anything else from this book, this mantra will help you quite a bit. As I said, we're going to give you special training in being prepared for questions, but I'll also provide you with everything else you will need to secure an acceptance offer from your next interview!

As you'll see in the answers I provide for you, I have highlighted the Qualities that the answer is emphasizing. You should now be familiar with what Qualities are and their importance in the tailoring process. The Qualities are noted in italics.

Also, be on the lookout for Multipliers. These are extra bits of information that supercharge your answer. They will be highlighted in bold. Remember, these answers are just guidelines. Every applicant has her own set of Qualities to infuse into these answers, so not everyone will answer the question in the same way.

Each question also has a **DO** and **DON'T** section that explores in depth what you should be aware of when faced with that type of question.

But before you run off with this section and start memorizing it, I'd like to interject yet another word of warning. **Remember: Each situation is different, just like every PA school interview is different.** *These are possible questions with suggested answers. They are not the magic key to the door of all knowledge or the pill to swallow to become the master of all interviews.*

Yes, this book is good—*really* good. It's based on my twenty-plus years of knowledge working with thousands of PA school applicants applying to programs across the United States. It is also based on my own experience on the ADCOM at Yale's PA program. *But it's still just a tool.* It's up to *you* to make this book work for you, and that means taking the time to really read through these Q&As, and then tailor them to fit your experiences and situations. Don't just memorize these and then spit them back like some sort of robot. You want to be accepted for who *you* are!

Now, on to the questions and answers!

TRADITIONAL QUESTIONS

Tell me about yourself.

You may see this question asked in a separate way: *Why are you a good fit for the PA profession?*

This question is the mother of all interview questions. I guarantee you will be asked this question at your interview, and, trust me, the committee doesn't want to know that you love to meditate on the beach at sunrise, or that you're an avid runner. What they're really asking is: *Why are you a good fit for our program and the PA profession?*

Your answer to this question can greatly influence the outcome of your interview. The interviewer wants to know that you have the necessary Qualities to fulfill exactly what they're looking for, the Perfect Applicant.

When answering this question, you'll want to weave a story that explains how your experiences and skillset have led you to the PA profession, and their program. Show them that you have the Qualities they're looking for.

Here is a good answer that will help guide you and help you build your own responses.

EXAMPLE ANSWER

I have been in the medical field for the past five years. My most recent experience is as a paramedic in a large urban community. **One reason I particularly enjoy this job, and the challenges that go with it, is the opportunity to connect with my patients, often in a significantly vulnerable time of their life.** In my current job, **I formed some significant patient relationships**, resulting in a deeper understanding of what it takes to be a competent medical provider.

My real strength is my ability to put my patients at ease. I pride myself on my reputation for being a **team player**. **When I commit to**

a job, I make sure I can be trusted to do my part to gain the trust of my coworkers.

What I am looking for now is a profession that values diversity, compassion, and life-long learning, where I can use my qualities and strengths to become a competent physician assistant.

QUALITIES

▶ Medical experience
▶ Ability to connect with patients
▶ Collaboration with coworkers
▶ Compassion
▶ Diversity
▶ Life-long learner

DO...

✓ Focus on the strengths that PA programs are looking for.
✓ Keep the story succinct and to the point.
✓ Keep the story focused on work accomplishments and qualities.

DON'T...

✘ Don't talk about your love for hiking or your passion for playing tennis.
✘ Don't stray.
✘ Don't focus on personal situations.
✘ Don't recount any situation that occurred over ten years ago.
✘ Don't talk about educational or work experiences that are not relevant to being a strong PA school applicant.
✘ Don't start with, "My name is..."

Why do you want to become a PA?

Ah, the million-dollar question! You better know the answer to this question like you know your social security number. *You will be asked this question!* Your answer should be your "elevator pitch." An elevator pitch is a term used in sales to make your case in three minutes as to why someone should invest in the product you're selling. Many times, a salesperson will walk into a client's office on a sales call and the client will say, "I'm very busy, but I'll give you three minutes." The salesperson will present the qualities and benefits of her product in three minutes to make the sale. The goal of your elevator pitch is to hit all your qualities, and the *benefits to the program* if they accept you. Make the interviewer's job easy by demonstrating that you have everything they're looking for in a student for their program.

Although you are not selling a product, you are selling yourself, right? Imagine you get into an elevator, and inside is the Dean of the PA program. You strike up a conversation, watching her pick the twelfth floor. She then asks you, "Why do you want to become a PA?" By the time you get to the twelfth floor, you better have answered the question. You need to have a well-prepared elevator pitch. I am always amused when I ask applicants, "So, why do you want to be a PA?" during a mock interview and their eyes widen; they start stuttering as if they didn't think this question was coming. You're applying to PA school, so of course they're going to ask you why you want to become a PA!

EXAMPLE ANSWER

First off, let me say that I know PA school, and working as a PA, will be challenging and will require specialized qualities and skills. Although I can't tell you that I know what it's like to be a PA, I can tell you that I believe I've acquired the qualities, skills, and experience necessary to qualify for your program and to be an effective, practicing PA in the future.

For instance, I have **persistence, dedication, and I'm a team player**. In college, I made the gymnastics team as a walk-on. I hadn't competed in gymnastics for a few years, and although I made the team, I did not compete my freshman year. I did compete in the next three years, and through sheer **dedication, hard work, and passion**

I eventually ended up as captain of a championship team my senior year.

In addition to being a team player, I am **community-oriented**. I grew up on a Navajo Indian Reservation, where I had several opportunities to give back. I **organized** Girl Scout and church projects in the community. I later **tutored friends and peers** in high school and college. And, I worked in "Upward Bound," a federally funded educational program that came about from the federal opportunity Act of 1964, which was also called the "War on Poverty Program."

On the reservation, there was only one, two-room clinic. If we needed anything but routine care, we had to travel hours to the nearest modern healthcare facility. Many of our people simply dealt with chronic pain from issues that could have been prevented if healthcare was more accessible.

With my fervent desire to work in healthcare and return to my community, I quit my job and immediately returned to school full-time. I began taking all the prerequisites necessary to gain acceptance into a PA program. I began working with mentally ill patients—a significant population of medically underserved people right here on our reservation. I began volunteering at a hospital near my college and picked up extra shifts in various departments.

My goal is to return home in a newly enhanced role as a PA, and continue serving my community. It is here that I feel I can make a significant difference in quality of healthcare on our reservation.

QUALITIES

- ▶ Persistence
- ▶ Dedication
- ▶ Team player
- ▶ Hard worker
- ▶ Passion
- ▶ Community oriented
- ▶ Leadership
- ▶ Service

DO...

✓ List as many qualities as you can relative to presenting yourself as an excellent candidate for PA school.

✓ Show the committee that you've done your homework and make it easy for them to choose you as a perfect fit for the PA profession.

✓ Demonstrate your qualities with examples, not just talk.

✓ Practice your elevator pitch until you can recite it in your sleep.

DON'T...

✗ Don't think, for one minute, that you will not be asked this question.

✗ Don't look shocked when asked this question.

✗ Don't forget to prepare your elevator pitch.

Why should we select you?
(Explain what you would bring to our program?)

This is a very common PA school interview question: *Why should we select you over the other applicants interviewing today? What makes you unique?* The interviewer will usually tell you how competitive the applicant pool is this year, and that they have a lot of qualified applicants to choose from. You might feel a little disheartened when you here this question, but don't let it get to you; it's not personal. If you weren't one of those highly qualified applicants, you wouldn't be there. The committee simply wants you to convince them that you have what it takes to be a god fit for their program.

Your goal at the interview is to show the committee that you are the solution to their problem, the Perfect Applicant.

EXAMPLE ANSWER

I believe that I am uniquely qualified to attend Stanford's PA program because of your program's mission to have its graduates focus on primary care in California, and to work in underserved communities.

I also know that it is important at Stanford to increase the enrollment and deployment of under-represented minorities. As you can see from my CASPA application**, I have several years of hands-on medical experience working in underserved communities**, and it seems to me that *Stanford Medical School's Free-Clinics, that provide quality healthcare to underserved populations,* is a testament to that commitment. There are so many PA programs that desire applicants to work in underserved areas, but few of them provide the opportunity to do this on campus. My experience working with underserved populations prepares me to hit the ground running in this program.

QUALITY

▶ Working in underserved areas

MULTIPLIER

▶ Stanford Medical School's Free Clinics

DO...

✓ Show you understand the mission of the program because you have researched their website, Google results, Facebook page, and YouTube channel.

✓ Research the program before going to the interview to show how you can best "fit in" with the culture.

✓ Show that you have experience working in underserved areas—that you don't just talk-the-talk, you walk-the-walk.

DON'T...

✗ Don't mention that you spoke with the other applicants before the interview and you feel that you are the most qualified.

✗ Don't brag.

✗ Don't be afraid to reiterate portions of your CASPA application that show you fit their needs.

✗ Don't bring up working in underserved areas if you have no experience doing so. Choose a different quality to focus on.

What is your greatest weakness?

Please do not say that you are a perfectionist or any other of those faux weaknesses that can be turned into strengths. And certainly, don't tell them that you're an alcoholic, but you are now in recovery. (If they hand you a rope, don't hang yourself with it.) This is a serious question that requires a serious answer. The committee wants to know what areas you've struggled with and what you've done to overcome these shortcomings. To answer this question appropriately, you will have to do a great deal of self-reflection. We all have weaknesses and turn them into positives that work for us; it shows adaptability, as well as providing insight into our character—two desirable traits to have as a PA student.

Beware: Interviewers also may be looking for flaws that fit a pattern of those applicants who may have dropped out of the program in the past.

EXAMPLE ANSWER

I tend to be a great starter and a poor finisher when it comes to writing papers. However, I've now learned a different approach to dealing with this issue. For example, when writing papers in college, I would always leave the most difficult, time consuming research for last, which led to procrastination and anxiety. Now, I've learned that **I do much better when I tackle the difficult research first**, while I have the most energy, and leave the less time-consuming research until the end, so I won't feel so burdened and panicky closer to the due date. **I break the project into smaller goals and set a deadline for achieving each one.**

I know as a student in this program, there is no time for procrastinating. Students cannot afford to fall behind in classwork. **I pride myself on being able to examine problems and come up with strategic solutions.**

QUALITIES

▶ Problem solver
▶ Goal oriented
▶ Critical thinking

DO...

✓ Turn a weakness into a strength.
✓ Spend some time reflecting on a legitimate weakness you've identified, and how you overcame it.
✓ Make sure you let them know that your weakness never gets in the way of your performance, and that you know how to strategically correct problems when they do arise.

DON'T...

✗ Don't tell the committee that you walk on water and have no weaknesses.
✗ Don't use a clichéd, faux weakness that can be turned into a strength; "I tend to pay too much attention to detail..."
✗ Don't hang yourself; now is not the time to talk about your alcoholism, arrest record, or the fact that you are a loner.

How would your friends describe you?

This question may catch you off-guard because it asks about the non-professional side of your life. The committee asks this question intentionally to see who you really are outside of your job or school. Remember to focus on the key attributes of making a great PA school student.

EXAMPLE ANSWER

I think my friends would describe me as a person who is an effective communicator. I am a great listener, and, therefore, **take the time to understand the other person's point of view**. As a result, I can be more empathetic and focus in on what the person is genuinely trying to communicate. As a medical assistant, patients frequently confide in me about their concerns relative to the reason for their appointments, or even issues going on in their personal lives. I listen to what they say, often repeat it back to them, and they feel that they've been heard. Through my work as a medical assistant, I've come to realize that **listening is an important trait, probably more than speaking is**.

QUALITIES

▶ Empathetic
▶ Effective listener
▶ Communication skills

DO...

✓ Try to tie in character traits that allow the listener to see you as an effective PA. Listening skill are essential to be an effective communicator, which are very important to gain the trust of patients.
✓ This interviewee has shown that she is an effective listener by using an example from a real-life situation: her job as a medical assistant.

DON'T...

✗ Don't describe traits that you cannot substantiate with an example.
✗ Don't choose character traits that are not in "sync" with those of the PA profession, or the qualities that the program desires in their students. Don't tell the committee that you like to isolate yourself, or that you like to party.
✗ Don't name more than three traits; you may not have the time to substantiate all of them.

What are your goals as a PA?

This question can be a trap to see if you plan to work in a primary care setting, work with underserved populations, or if your goals are inconsistent with the program's mission. To make this question easy to answer, I advise that you break the goals down into short, medium, and long-term goals.

EXAMPLE ANSWER

I have short, medium, and long-range goals once I become a PA.

My short-term goal is to work, clinically, in the primary care setting with underserved populations. I wish to build on what I've learned in PA school and **solidify a strong foundation in medicine** that will help me throughout my entire career.

My medium-range goal—say, five years from now—is to work in research. I worked on a lot of research projects in college and I have a strong desire to continue to do so as a physician assistant. *I notice that City College has done some groundbreaking research in areas like PTSD, Alzheimer's, and developing a new aspirin to fight cancer.* I have a personal interest in finding a cure for Alzheimer's disease.

My long-term goal is to tie in my clinical background, along with my research experiences, and **one day teach at a PA program. I would like to give back to the profession** by helping to educate and motivate students.

QUALITIES

▶ Goal-oriented
▶ Desire to work with underserved populations
▶ Give back to the profession

MULTIPLIER

▶ City College's groundbreaking research in PTSD, Alzheimer's, and developing a new aspirin

DO...

✓ Include a supercharger: The groundbreaking research conducted at the program.

✓ Break you goals into short, medium, and long-term goals.

✓ Research the program. The applicant has done her homework and has also tied her answer into the fact that she has a history of doing research in the past.

✓ Support your answer with a specific example found in your research that the admissions committee will not expect you to know about. In the example above, this is their "groundbreaking research."

✓ Include three acceptable scenarios in your answer, which could include practicing clinical medicine (especially in primary care), doing research, and teaching at a PA program.

DON'T...

✗ Don't tell the admissions committee that you want to start your career in a specialty, like cardiology. This goal is inconsistent with the mission of the program and it shows that you are close-minded with respect to discovering opportunities in the other disciplines you will encounter on clinical rotations.

✗ Don't forget to research the program before your interview.

✗ Don't discuss anything specific that you cannot support on your CASPA application. If you have never done research, don't tell the committee that doing research is one of your goals, unless you can provide strong justification for this decision.

✗ Don't start out by saying, "I want to graduate, and pass my boards, then..." Listen to the question! The question is about your goals as a PA, not a student. Why would you take your boards again?

Why do you want to attend *our* program?

Why do you want to attend Quinnipiac's PA program? This question requires an answer that is specific to Quinnipiac's program, and not an answer that could be used for *any* program. You want to use specifics that you've learned in your research on the program and try to incorporate some Multipliers to give you an edge over the average applicant who has not done her homework. The admissions committee will be evaluating you to see if Quinnipiac is your first choice, or if you're using this interview to hedge your chances of getting accepted elsewhere. The more specific you are relative to Quinnipiac's program, the more likely you are to convince the committee that you truly plan to attend their program if you're accepted. This is where supercharging your answer will set you apart from the crowd.

EXAMPLE ANSWER

There are some obvious reasons why I want to attend Quinnipiac. Your **first-time pass-fail rate on the PANCE is currently ninety-eight percent over the past five years**. I know if I attend this program I will be well prepared to pass my boards and become a certified PA. This program is **consistently ranked as one of the top-ten PA programs in the country by U.S. News & World Report**. The program has been **accredited since 1995**, and I know that if I attend this program I will benefit from a strong curriculum and well-established clinical rotation sites. Additionally, *Quinnipiac University has a new Center for Medicine designed for collaborative learning for students in medicine, nursing, and allied health, with over twenty-four teaching laboratories, including a cadaver lab.*

But the main reason I went to attend Quinnipiac is that your **program's vision aligns perfectly with why I want to be a PA in the first place**: to provide high quality affordable healthcare that is accessible to everyone in the community, and an **emphasis on**

working with diverse populations. I know that Quinnipiac is in a suburb of New Haven, Connecticut, a place where there is plenty of opportunity to accomplish this vision, and **my five years of experience working as an X-ray technician at Harlem Hospital will allow me to carry out this vision in a newly enhanced role**.

QUALITY
▶ Prepared
▶ Aligned vision
▶ Diversity
▶ Medical experience

MULTIPLIER
▶ New "Center for Medicine"

DO...
✓ Know the critical information about the program: first-time pass-fail rate on the boards, longevity of the program, vision, mission, and facilities (cadaver lab).
✓ Study the program's website to see if their vision aligns with your goals.
✓ Start the second paragraph with, "But the main reason I want to attend Quinnipiac..." This statement specifically answers the question, "Why Quinnipiac (out of all the other programs)?"
✓ Include examples from your own experiences.
✓ Search the website for any information that will set you apart from the other applicants.
✓ Break this answer into two paragraphs: The first paragraph simply lists multiple favorable facts about the program (which can apply to 200 other programs), the second paragraph gets specific about why *this* program, as opposed to the many other programs in the country that also have longevity and high PANCE rates.

DON'T...

- ✘ Don't give a generalized answer that is not specific to the program where you are interviewing.
- ✘ Don't forget to scan every page of the program's website, Facebook page, Google results, and YouTube channel, looking for *supercharged* information.
- ✘ Don't simply rely on the statistics of the program to use for your answer. Provide a "main reason" for applying there.

Which program is your top choice?

Always a tricky question. If you name a different program than the one you're currently interviewing with, you risk the chance of offending the committee and being rejected. However, if you name the program you're interviewing with as your top choice, you risk the chance of coming across as being disingenuous, or even lying if the program is obviously *not*, in fact, your top choice. This is one of those questions where I advise to answer the question without *really* answering the question. After all, the wrong answer to this question can be the kiss of death for your chances of acceptance.

EXAMPLE ANSWER

When choosing PA programs that I was interested in applying to, **I selected those schools where I felt my background was a good fit for the program**, as well as programs that met criteria I felt were important to getting an excellent education. I feel that I am a good fit for this program, and that **this program meets all the criteria I am looking for to get a quality education and prepare me to become a competent PA**.

QUALITY

- ▶ Researched programs for "fit"
- ▶ Developed a common denominator for choosing programs

DO...

✓ Research programs where your background and qualifications are a good fit.

✓ Decide upon a common denominator that you'll use to decide which programs you'll apply to. These could be PANCE rates, access to a cadaver lab, international rotations, commitment to underserved communities, etc.

✓ Be prepared to discuss these common denominators if asked why you chose the programs you have.

DON'T...

✗ Don't mention geography as a reason to choose their program. Choosing a program strictly because it's close to where you live, is not going to go over well with the interviewer and it could be an insult to the committee.

✗ Don't mention *another* program as your top choice; it's too risky. Use the technique above to give a generalized, non-specific answer.

How have you stayed current and informed on the PA profession?

Are you well informed about the PA profession? This question is designed to see if you are a serious applicant, or just testing the waters. The PA profession is a desirable one with regards to job outlook, pay, and prestige. Serious applicants will invest the time learning about the PA profession and stay current on issues and policies affecting it. Those applicants who are not serious about becoming a PA, or who are not applying for the right reasons, will expend the least amount of time and energy doing research. These applicants are quickly weeded out by seasoned admissions committee members.

EXAMPLE ANSWER

I stay current and informed about the PA profession through **my membership with the American Academy of Physician Assistants (AAPA), my membership in my state chapter of the AAPA**, reading the Journal of the American Academy of Physician Assistants (JAAPA), and by shadowing PAs in the field.

Since **I am a veteran**, I was pleased to read that **the AAPA is a partner with the "Joining Forces Campaign."** The campaign is involved in the important mission to support U.S. service members, veterans, and those who have fallen. The PA profession began with a class of former navy corpsman, and it's good to see that those military roots are still important today.

In my home state of Florida, PAs participate in **Legislative Days in Tallahassee**, and provide information to state legislators by relating the importance of the team approach to health care, and how PAs can assist in increasing access to care for all Floridians. The PAs who attend also discuss the limitations that keep PAs from practicing to the full extent of their education, training, and experience.

In an article I read in the latest edition of JAAPA, I learned that in November 2015, **the NCCPA proposed a new recertification process for the PA profession**. The NCCPA has sent out questionnaires to get feedback from practicing PAs about their thoughts on the proposed new certification practice. They found that the three most common practice areas were family practice/general practice, surgical subspecialties, and emergency medicine.

I find this information interesting and useful, as **I consider myself a lifelong learner and I am passionate about joining the PA profession**. I now know that I have these great resources to help me keep abreast of current events and issues that are currently in the news.

QUALITIES

▶ Member of the AAPA and her state chapter of the AAPA
▶ Military veteran
▶ Lifelong learner
▶ Passion for the PA profession

MULTIPLIER

▶ Joining Forces Campaign
▶ Legislative Days in Tallahassee
▶ NCCPA's proposed new recertification process

DO...

✓ Join the AAPA, your state chapter of the AAPA, and read JAAPA.
✓ Choose an article from each on current events happening in the PA profession, and be prepared to speak about the issue.
✓ Explain how you believe these current events and issues will impact the profession.

DON'T...

✗ Don't come to the interview unprepared to talk about current events and issues facing the PA profession.
✗ Don't be lazy! Do your homework before the interview.

What do you think is the biggest challenge you'll face as a PA?

Are you aware of the challenges PAs face on a daily basis? By asking this question, the interviewer is trying to see if you've paid attention to these issues while shadowing PAs.

EXAMPLE ANSWER

From my shadowing experiences, and from many discussions with PAs, I feel the most challenging part of the profession is

having to explain the role of the PA to many patients who are expecting to see the "doctor." Patients frequently ask, "You mean you're a medical assistant?"

One PA I shadowed, Marissa, explained to me that over the course of her twenty-year career as a PA, she has been asked this question frequently—although much less frequently now. She explained that it used to frustrate her to have to explain the difference between a PA and a MA daily. **She tells me that she now reframes the question, and sees it not as a challenge, but as an opportunity to educate patients about the PA profession.** The result has been an increased awareness about the PA profession and the understanding of PAs as competent healthcare professionals.

QUALITY
▶ Understanding of the PA profession
▶ Turning a negative into a positive

DO...
✓ Ask a lot of questions when you shadow PAs relative to the challenges they encounter in the profession.
✓ Ask patients that you come across, either while shadowing or through your current job in healthcare, what their thoughts are about being seen by a PA.
✓ Try to reframe your answer and turn it into an opportunity.

DON'T...
✗ Don't speak poorly of the MA profession, or any other practitioners.
✗ Don't become defensive.
✗ Don't criticize the profession.

If you had a patient with a language barrier, how would you assist that patient?

Do you have effective communication skills? Being able to communicate with patients is a necessity when it comes to taking a medical history and discussing a treatment plan. If there is a communication barrier between provider and patient, it is the provider's responsibility to find a solution to this problem. You will encounter such situations many times in your career as a PA.

EXAMPLE ANSWER

In my job as a medical assistant, I often interact with patients who speak a foreign language exclusively, or have limited English speaking skills. **I utilize several approaches to ease communication problems.**

The first thing I would do is to see if there are any family members in the waiting room, or if any of our staff members speak the same language as the patient.

If not, the next thing I would do is **slow down while speaking, and continue to ask questions, understanding that patients have various levels of fluency. I will also use nonverbal communication; like charts on the wall, pictures, or by writing on the exam paper.**

Additionally, **I find that having patience and maintaining a sense of humor can sometimes put the patient at ease and make communication less stressful.** Many times, I find that patients can speak the language, but become embarrassed to do so in public. A little patience and humor can go a long way in these situations.

I like to keep communication personal, but if all else failed, I would use one of the new translation apps on my cell phone to ensure the patient comprehends everything I am saying. I would also advise the patient to bring a translator with her to the next visit to overcome the communication obstacle and make our communication more personal.

QUALITIES

- ▶ Communication skills
- ▶ Ingenuity
- ▶ Compassion
- ▶ Empathy
- ▶ Thinking outside the box

DO...

- ✓ Know your staff and the languages they speak to translate, if necessary.
- ✓ Provide a list of three or four techniques you use to communicate with patients who do not speak English.
- ✓ Mention an example of a patient you worked with who did not speak English.
- ✓ Start out with as much personal communication as possible, and go up the latter to technology, if needed.

DON'T...

- ✗ Don't mention frustration in this situation.
- ✗ Don't tell the committee you've never encountered this situation.
- ✗ Don't forget to prepare for this question!

What is your biggest strength?

Besides "Tell me about yourself," and "Why do you want to be a PA?", this question is one of the most commonly asked during any interview. Be prepared for this question. Think of several strengths that you have (relative to the qualities of a PA) and keep your answer brief, honest, and to the point. Be sure you can back up that strength with an example.

EXAMPLE ANSWER

As an office manager for a large medical practice, **I had to learn all phases of clinical and administrative management, from developing work flow procedures, to supervising medical assistants, to handling billing issues. I can multi-task and I have a cooperative style.** I am also able to delegate tasks effectively and gain the confidence and cooperation of coworkers. **I was voted "employee of the year" two years in a row.**

QUALITIES

▶ Organized
▶ Ability to multi-task
▶ Self-starter
▶ Cooperative style
▶ "Employee of the year"

DO...

✓ Tie your experience to the needs and desires of the PA profession.
✓ Mention any awards you may have won, like "employee of the year."
✓ Give a brief answer that gets right to the point and demonstrates your ability to get along well with others.

DON'T...

✗ Don't brag.
✗ Don't forget to prepare, so that you don't draw a blank and come up clueless.
✗ Don't make claims you can't back up with facts.
✗ Don't be overly modest, but don't inflate your answer either.
✗ Don't name a strength that does not pertain to the qualities required of a strong PA school applicant/PA.

Why do you want to change careers?

EXAMPLE ANSWER

For thirteen years I worked in advertising. In December of 2011, while attending the equivalent of the Academy Awards for advertising, **I received three gold "Addy's" and two Silver "Addy's" for my accomplishments in advertising.** Although I should have been excited and proud, I had never felt so unfulfilled in my life. During that event, I recalled the goal I had set twenty-three years earlier, which was to pursue a career in medicine.

As a Grey advertising account executive, **I could expand my leadership and soft skills. As the liaison between agency and client, I managed multiple projects from inception to completion, often in high-pressure and time-sensitive situations. I also became very adept at translating and presenting ideas and strategies to clients**, and I found myself naturally comfortable working with senior executives and **diverse teammates. I enjoyed participating in teams and working with diverse individuals** who possessed a broad assortment of skills. Together, we produced great products for our clients, while also achieving company goals.

But, I now yearned to get back on the path toward working in healthcare, and I decided to pursue that goal I had twenty-three years earlier. **I felt that the skills I learned as an account executive were transferable to that of a healthcare provider.** I believe the skills that I have developed parallel those of a physician assistant.

I gave up my high paying job as an account executive, **enrolled back into college to meet the prerequisites classes to attend PA school, and began volunteering as a physical therapy aid, a nurses' aid, and a patient advocate at Shepherd's Clinic. I also began shadowing several PAs, joined the American Academy of Physician Assistants and my state chapter of the AAPA, read JAAPA frequently, and did as much research as I could on the PA profession, including specific research on this program.** I believe that throughout my journey in life, I've acquired the skills and qualities necessary to become a competent and compassionate PA.

QUALITIES

- ▶ Accomplished
- ▶ Leadership
- ▶ Transferable skills
- ▶ Ability to multi-task
- ▶ Ability to handle stress
- ▶ Motivation to become a PA
- ▶ Community service
- ▶ Passion

DO...

- ✓ Mention any transferable skills that would be valuable as a PA student/PA.
- ✓ Explain your motivation for making the career change.
- ✓ List what you've done to prepare yourself for a career as a PA.
- ✓ Show that you've done your homework on the PA profession.

DON'T...

- ✗ Don't mention being fired from your last job.
- ✗ Don't talk negatively about your last career.
- ✗ Don't talk about better pay or more opportunity.

What is the difference between a PA and a nurse practitioner?

Due to the predicted shortages and maldistribution of diverse types of healthcare providers, the consensus for demand for healthcare services is on the rise. Therefore, NPs and PAs are going to play a major role in the future. The question being asked is if you understand the differences and similarities between the two professions. There is a significant area of overlap between NPs and PAs. There are a couple of ways to go about answering this question: focus on the differences or focus on the similarities in the profession.

I believe there is also an underlying motive for asking this question: Do you have a bias against nurse practitioners? Many applicants will talk about how PAs are trained in the "medical model" and nurse practitioners are trained in the "nursing model," yet have no idea what those mean. Applicants will also discuss the dependent nature of the PA profession and the independent nature of the nurse practitioner profession. I suggest that you take a different approach to this question if you want to stand out from the crowd.

EXAMPLE ANSWER

There are some obvious differences between the PA and NP professions. In many states, NPs are independent practitioners, and, currently, PAs are dependent practitioners, which may change when Full Practice Authority and Responsibility (FPAR) becomes the law nationwide.

Additionally, you must first be a nurse before you can become a nurse practitioner. PAs come from a variety of backgrounds in the medical field. Nurse practitioner students train at nursing programs, while many times PA students train at medical schools, or at least in the fast track model patterned after medical students during World War II.

However, through my experience shadowing PAs, and working in a large clinic as a medical assistant, I've come to realize that **there are more similarities than differences between the two professions**. Both PAs and nurse practitioners are mid-level practitioners who work toward the same goal of treating patients to the best of their ability. In fact, I believe that if everyone in our clinic covered their name tags, the patients wouldn't know if they were a PA, physician, or nurse practitioner. **We are all on the same team and have a common goal: providing the best care to the patient.**

QUALITIES
▶ Thorough understanding of both professions
▶ Shows no bias toward the NP profession (inclusive)

DO...

✓ Demonstrate that you understand the basic differences between PAs and NPs: in the training, education, and requirements for each profession.

✓ Be inclusive; discuss the similarities, as well as the differences, to show that you aren't biased against your future colleagues.

✓ Stress the fact that we are all on the same team, looking out for the patient and not focused on our differences.

DON'T...

✗ Don't speak negatively about nurse practitioners.

✗ Don't talk about the medical model or the nursing model unless asked.

✗ Don't talk about the "holistic" approach that NPs learn in school. Many applicants with whom I do mock interviews talk about the nursing model but can't explain exactly what the nursing model is!

What do you do in your spare time?
(Tell us about something that's not already in your application.)

This seemingly "soft" question is asked to see how well you will match the program's needs and goals. Be sure your answer includes a quality.

EXAMPLE ANSWER

I like to play softball in the summer and basketball in the winter. However, my true passion is working on my condominium's beautification project. I created and lead a group of condo owners to make it our mission to be *the* most beautiful condo units in town. So far, we've gone on to plant over a hundred trees and multiple flower beds. **I love organizing, inspiring and working together with my neighbors to make our community a better place to live.**

QUALITIES
- ▶ Leadership
- ▶ Team player
- ▶ Inspiring

DO...
- ✓ The admissions committee isn't really interested in your personal life; they just want to know that you are a balanced person with a lot of diverse interests and activities.
- ✓ Describe hobbies and pastimes that relate to the qualities of being a great PA. If you like volunteering for retreats at your church, helping people and communities around the country or in foreign countries, be sure to mention that you are a team player, empathetic, and willing to sacrifice for others.
- ✓ Stay up-to-date on current events in the PA profession.

DON'T...
- ✗ Don't name hobbies or interests that are not relevant to the qualities of being a PA student or a PA-C.
- ✗ Don't tell the interviewer that you are actually a couch potato and enjoy sitting home alone watching movies.

Is there anything else we should know about you?

The interviewer is giving you a chance to make a good impression, while at the same time, searching for any disqualifying factors that may come up. Be honest, but keep skeletons in the closet where they belong. Everyone makes mistakes, but unless your mistakes are going to affect your interview, keep them to yourself. Instead, find something about you that is interesting and can be used to relate to another strength that would be relevant to PA school. Don't mention that you have a history of domestic violence and your ex-spouse has a restraining order on you. Keep it positive and keep it business-like.

EXAMPLE ANSWER

I didn't mention an interesting anecdote when I was a safety manager at one of my jobs with a construction company. I had just completed my CPR and First Aid courses, and a man on the site suddenly went into cardiac arrest. My foreman looked at me and said, "You're in charge of safety!" I had practiced on a dummy but never on a live person. I knew I had to keep calm and simply do what I was taught. I began reviving him while others called 911. He survived, and later thanked me for saving his life. I know that as a PA, these types of situations will likely happen in the future. **I learned that keeping calm and putting one's training into motion will always help resolve a critical situation.**

QUALITY

▶ Ability to remain calm under pressure

DO...

✓ Choose a memorable closing story that casts you in a favorable light and will stay with the interviewer long after you leave. Of course, you cannot and should not make something up, but think of a time when you acted well under pressure, especially since PA school requires that quality.

✓ Relate any answers to this question to PA school.

DON'T...

✗ Don't shrug helplessly as if you hadn't a clue.

✗ Don't answer with a flat out "No."

✗ Don't spill your guts!

HYPOTHETICAL QUESTIONS

If you could be a color/animal/tree/fruit, what would it be, and why?

When I sat on the admissions committee at Yale's PA program, we rarely asked hypothetical questions. However, during my many years coaching thousands of PA school applicants interviewing at various programs around the country, many of them reported back to me about their frustration with answering hypothetical questions like "If you were a color, what would it be and why?" Applicants complain, "What if I choose blue as a color versus green?" and "What do these questions have to do with getting into PA school?"

At first, I could not figure out why these questions were asked either. So, I did my research, and believe it or not, the answers to these questions perfectly drive home the point of infusing *Qualities* into your answers at your interview.

You should approach these questions as a way for the admissions committee to gain insight into your personality and, most of all, your Qualities. *Remember: It's not about you, it's about them.* Your answer should reflect the fact that you have the Qualities they're looking for in a PA school applicant. Your answers should focus on Qualities; the more creative you are, the better.

Remember, there are no right or wrong answers to these questions. It's all about trying to evaluate your thought process, how you handle being put on the spot, and your ability to be creative. Do not overthink these questions.

I will list the DOs and DON'Ts for any of these questions first:

DO...
✓ Infuse at least two Qualities into your answer.
✓ Practice with these types of questions before your interview.
✓ Be creative.

DON'T...

- ✖ Don't respond, "Green, because it's my favorite color" or "A dog, because dogs are man's best friend." *It's not about you, it's about them.*
- ✖ Don't say, "Hmm, I never thought about that."

If you were a color, what would it be, and why?

Use colors that highlight your best qualities, and don't forget to justify your answer.

EXAMPLE ANSWER

I would be charcoal grey. Charcoal grey is a **unique** color, it reminds me of **professionalism, and it blends well with other colors**.

QUALITIES

- ▶ Unique applicant
- ▶ Professionalism
- ▶ Team player

If you were a tree, what would it be, and why?

EXAMPLE ANSWER

I would be a palm tree. In the worst of storms, a palm tree will bend to the ground and not break, and after the storm it will pop right back up. A palm tree is very **flexible and very resilient**.

QUALITIES

- ▶ Flexible
- ▶ Resilient

If you were a fruit, what would it be and why?

EXAMPLE ANSWER

I would be a banana. **A banana is a very substantial fruit, and it blends well in a fruit salad.**

QUALITIES

▶ Substance
▶ Team player

If you were an animal, what would it be and why?

EXAMPLE ANSWER

I would be an eagle. An eagle can fly ten-thousand feet above the ground and see for miles and miles around. An eagle can also focus in on the tiniest animal on the desert floor. **An eagle can see the big picture, as well as focus in on the smallest details.**

QUALITIES

▶ Ability to see the big picture
▶ Pay attention to details

If you could have dinner with anyone living or dead who would it be and why?

EXAMPLE ANSWER

I would choose Dr. Eugene Stead, the founder of the PA profession. I would like to discuss his decision to start up the PA profession and ask him if he ever envisioned that it would grow to the extent it has. I would ask him about his thoughts on Full Practice Authority and Responsibility. I would ask him what, if anything, he'd like to see changed in the profession right now, and finally, **I would thank him for the foresight he had when starting the PA profession.**

QUALITIES

▶ Gratitude

DO...

✓ Think about a person who has many qualities that are relevant to becoming a great PA.

✓ Discuss why you would choose this person.

DON'T...

✗ Don't choose a person that does not possess the qualities that are needed to become a great PA.

✗ Don't choose superheroes or movie stars because you personally like them. It's not about you, it's about them. Do you need super powers to become a PA?

Is there anything else we should know about you?

Your interviewer is not only allowing you to make a good impression, she is also looking to see if you mention any disqualifying factors. Be honest, but this is not the time to talk about any skeletons in your closet. For instance, you wouldn't want to tell her that you like to party on the weekends with your friends. The admissions committee knows that everyone makes mistakes, but if those mistakes are going to affect your chances of getting accepted to the program, keep them to yourself. Find something interesting about yourself that can be used to relate another strength to the program/profession. Keep it positive and keep it focused on the program/profession.

EXAMPLE ANSWER

I didn't mention that I was a former Navy hospital corpsman. My first assignment was with the U.S. Marine Corps as a field corpsman for a company of front-line marines. When we initially arrived at the base, all the corpsman had to complete another six weeks of training in field medicine. We would periodically do week-long field exercises in the swamps of Camp Lejeune, North Carolina. One evening, I heard a shout, "Corpsman up," which means somebody was hurt and they needed immediate medical attention. When I got to the scene, one of the marines was in cardiac arrest. The Gunnery Sargent said, "Doc, you're the corpsman!" I learned about CPR in hospital corps school and in field training, but I never had to use it. **I knew that I had to keep calm and simply do what I was taught. I revived him, while others called for a base ambulance.** Since I was a newbie, if you will, I knew that all eyes were on me to see how I handled this situation. I felt a lot of pressure. **I stayed calm and focused and put my training into motion to save this marine's life.** I think my experience in the navy was excellent training for a career as a physician assistant.

QUALITY

▶ Ability to remain calm under pressure

DO...

✓ Provide a memorable closing that casts you as the hero. This will leave a lasting impression on the committee or interviewer long after you leave the room.
✓ Relate your answer to the job of a physician assistant.

DON'T...

✗ Don't shrug helpless as if you haven't a clue
✗ Don't answer with a flat out "No."
✗ Don't spill your guts; this is not a time to talk about family drama, or at time when you got suspended from school.

What experience do you have that qualifies you to join our program?

Even if you are a non-traditional applicant, the committee is looking to see if you have the qualities needed to succeed in their PA program, and as a PA once you graduate. This is a fantastic opportunity for non-traditional applicants to demonstrate that they have transferable skills that relate to the PA profession.

EXAMPLE ANSWER

My first job after graduating college with a degree in chemistry was as a sales representative for a chemical company. **I worked autonomously** in the field selling chemicals for industrial water treatment, industrial boilers, and cooling towers. I was expected to use my **communication and presentation skills** to sell the chief engineers on our products, and on my ability to service the account. To properly service the boilers and cooling towers, I had to use my **analytical skills as a chemist to diagnose and solve problems**. Properly maintaining these large pieces of equipment meant the difference between losing a great deal of money for the company, or saving a great deal of money. By doing an effective job, I was rewarded with increases in income, and the chief engineer was rewarded by his company for saving money. It was a win-win situation.

QUALITY

▶ Worked autonomously
▶ Communication skills
▶ Problem solver

DO...

✓ Relate your experiences to qualities that programs look for in strong applicants.
✓ Select a situation where you are the "hero."
✓ Focus on the benefits to everyone involved; "win-win"

DON'T...

✗ Don't babble about irrelevant material.
✗ Don't make it all about you.
✗ Don't feel the need to relate this answer to medicine.

Are you good at making decisions? Explain.

PAs consistently must make decisions daily. Some decisions can be critical ones. The interviewer wants to know if you have the skills necessary to do so.

EXAMPLE ANSWER

I do think I make good decisions, yes. There are always many ways to tackle a problem, and there is often a right way and a wrong way. In healthcare, providers cannot afford to make too many wrong decisions. That's why **I try never to make decisions out of emotion; especially anger, frustration, or fear**. If I am feeling a strong emotion, I will put off the decision until I can be more objective. **I will often consult with colleagues to get an objective opinion. I will also do some quick research in manuals or online to make an educated decision.** For example, after my company closed its doors and moved out of state, I was unemployed for a period, and I was forced to make some sacrifices. Unemployment was not providing enough money to pay the mortgage. I did the math and realized that **I had to let go of my emotional attachment to my house and sell it if I wanted to survive financially.**

QUALITIES

▶ Analytical thinking
▶ Research
▶ Humility

DO...

✓ Give a responsible answer that shows you know something about decision-making.
✓ Show that you've had to make some difficult decisions.
✓ Focus on the benefits to everyone involved.

DON'T...

✗ Don't answer with a simple "yes" or "no"
✗ Don't go off on a tangent.

Describe the role of the PA as you understand it.

Do you know what you are getting yourself into? Do you understand that the PA profession is currently a *dependent* one, and that you are not going to be in charge? Do you have a good working knowledge of what real PAs do on the job? Have you done your homework? Can you demonstrate that you have the qualities that would make a great PA? Are you knowledgeable on the topic of Full Practice Authority and Responsibility (FPAR), or Optimal Team Practice (OTP)? (If not, I strongly recommend that you learn about FPAR/OTP before your interview.)

EXAMPLE ANSWER

Physician Assistants are healthcare professionals licensed to practice medicine under the license of a supervising physician. PAs are considered mid-level practitioners; however, PAs work very autonomously in most practices. **The role of the PA** is to take a medical history and perform a medical examination. The PA will then compile a differential diagnosis, order the appropriate diagnostic tests, if needed, and prescribe a treatment plan. **PAs collaborate with their supervising physician, as well as medical specialists, and virtually every member of the healthcare team as appropriate.**

PAs currently can be found in almost every specialty area of medicine and surgery. PAs also enjoy the benefit of lateral movement; being able to change specialties during their career.

In 2017, PAs at the AAPA national convention voted to pursue Full Practice Authority and Responsibility. It could take a few years for FPAR to be implemented in every state. Once FPAR is fully integrated, the dependent nature of the PA profession will be eliminated.

QUALITIES

▶ Knowledge of the PA's role in healthcare
▶ Knowledge about the future role of PAs with the advent of FPAR

DO...

✓ Shadow several PAs to learn about the PA's role in the different specialty areas.

✓ Research the role of the PA online and through various forums.

✓ Join the American Academy of Physician Assistants (AAPA) and your state chapter of the AAPA to have a basic knowledge of issues facing the profession at the national and state level; FPAR.

✓ Keep your answer brief and generalized.

DON'T...

✗ Don't try to "wing it."

✗ Don't ignore the role/importance of shadowing PAs.

✗ Don't be complacent.

You mentioned earlier that you want to become a PA because you want to practice medicine, and that you want to help people. Why not become a nurse practitioner or a physician?

Why do you want to be a PA versus a physician or a nurse practitioner? The committee simply wants to see if you have a good understanding of each of the three professions and what your thought process is for choosing to be a PA. They may also be looking to see if you are using the PA profession as a stepping stone to eventually become a physician.

EXAMPLE ANSWER

I believe many PA school applicants probably thought about becoming a physician at one point or another. I know I did. A long time ago **I thought hard about which route I wanted to take to be able to practice medicine.** To become a physician, I would have to invest eight years of my life in medical school, both in the classroom and doing an internship and residency. If I wanted to specialize and do a fellowship, that would require another two years of training. Additionally, **I would acquire over $300,000 in debt** along the way and have **little time to start a family and be present**. Finally, **I would be locked into one specialty area**, and I wouldn't be able to change specialties without a significant amount of formal training.

I never considered becoming a nurse practitioner for one obvious reason: I'm not a nurse. I would have to enroll in a nursing program and spend three or four years studying to become a nurse. Then I would have to work in the field for a few years gaining clinical experience before applying to a nurse practitioner program. Then, I would have to spend another two years, or more, in a nurse practitioner program before I would be allowed to practice medicine. Again, for me, **becoming a nurse practitioner would be a much more significant investment of time and money than becoming a PA**.

I feel that **becoming a PA is the best opportunity for me to practice medicine. I could become a PA in approximately two years and begin practicing medicine immediately** after passing the PANCE. My student loan debt will be significantly less than the NP or MD route, and I will have much more time and **flexibility to raise a family** and pursue my other interests in life. Unlike a physician specialist, who typically remains in her chosen specialty for the entirety of her career, as a PA I would have more **flexibility and the opportunity for lateral movement, without having to invest a lot of time in formal training**.

QUALITY

▶ Thorough understanding of the PA profession
▶ Understands the differences between a physician and a nurse practitioner
▶ Reasoning skills
▶ Practicality

DO...

✓ Be honest. If you have considered becoming a physician, don't be afraid to say so. The committee will not hold this against you and will appreciate your honesty.

✓ Be prepared to discuss the differences between the three career fields.

✓ Show the rational approach you used to make your decision to become a PA.

✓ Finish with a strong, unequivocal reason why you eventually chose to pursue the PA profession over the others.

DON'T...

✗ Don't degrade the other two professions.

✗ Don't use the PA profession as a stepping stone to medical school; the committee will sense your motive.

✗ Don't lie. If you ever considered one of the other two career fields, admit it and justify why you chose to become a PA instead.

✗ Don't simply state why you want to become a PA and avoid discussing the other two professions.

✗ Don't be unprepared for this question.

Please tell us if you've applied to other programs, why you applied there, and which one is your number one choice?

Oh boy! Talk about anxiety. The interviewer is putting you on the spot in two ways; she's asking you to specifically name the other programs that you've applied to, and she wants to know if you get accepted to several programs, which is your number one choice. The interviewer also wants to see if you have a specific rationale, or common denominator, for choosing the programs you have. Many applicants feel a lot of anxiety when asked this question. "Will the interviewer know ahead of time if I have applied to other programs?" "Will the interviewer know which programs I applied to?" "What if this is *not* my number one choice?"

Don't worry, the interviewer expects that you've applied to multiple programs; you are motivated to become a PA, aren't you? Probably the most challenging part of answering this question is telling the interviewer if this program is your first choice or not. You must provide a convincing answer, and I'll show you how to do that.

EXAMPLE ANSWER

In addition to this program (Duke), I've applied to four other programs: The University of Iowa, Emory, George Washington, and Quinnipiac. All these programs are rated in the *U.S. News & World Report* as Top Ten PA programs in the country. All these programs offer a master's degree. All five meets or exceeds the national average first-time pass/fail rates on the PANCE. All five programs have been in existence for at least fifteen years, and Duke for over fifty-years.

Duke is my first choice. I have already been accepted to two other programs, and if either of those were my top choices, I would not be here today. There would be no reason to continue interviewing. Duke is the birthplace of the physician assistant profession, with a rich history of training some of the best physician assistants in the country. *I particularly like Duke's Common Problem Labs (CPLs) that offer unique opportunities for students to divide into small groups and discuss patient scenarios pertaining to a specific clinical unit.*

QUALITIES
▶ Research
▶ Honesty
▶ Decision making
▶ Preparedness

MULTIPLIER

▶ Common Problem Labs

DO...

✓ Be prepared for this question.

✓ Give your answer in the first sentence.

✓ Apply to more than one program; you don't want the interviewer to think that you are putting all your eggs in one basket. Additionally, if you only apply to one program, you apparently are not that motivated to become a PA.

✓ Look for a common thread amongst the programs you apply to.

✓ Have a method/ common denominator for choosing programs

✓ Look for a multiplier to explain your first-choice; it makes your answer much more credible.

DON'T...

✗ Don't lie. If you applied to more programs, list them.

✗ Don't tell the interviewer that her program is your number one choice without being able to back it up.

✗ Don't be inconsistent with the programs you choose; if you want a master's degree, don't select a community college program, or a bachelor's program.

✗ Don't tell the interviewer what you think she wants to hear, or you'll come off shallow and untrustworthy.

✗ Don't waffle on this question.

Can you tell me about your most memorable patient?

This question is meant to see if any of your patients have made an impact on you, and perhaps changed the way you think, or helped you become more empathetic and sympathetic. This question also gives you the opportunity to discuss some of the *soft skills* you may want to bring up.

EXAMPLE ANSWER

My most memorable patient was a fifteen-year-old boy named John. I was working as an emergency room technician, and John was brought in by EMS after being involved in an accident while riding his mini-bike. We immediately brought John into one of the major trauma rooms, transferred him to the exam table, and the physicians began to assess his injuries. It was obvious that John was in critical condition and was going to need immediate treatment if he was going to survive.

After only a few minutes, it was clear that John was probably not going to make it. He repeatedly went into cardiac arrest and had to be resuscitated several times. John's parents were right outside of the doors, and one of the physicians on the team advised them that John's prognosis was poor. We could hear the wailing from the hallway. "I told him not to take that mini-bike onto the street," his father shouted. It was heart-wrenching.

The team quickly realized that John was in cardiac tamponade, and decided the only hope was to open his chest immediately and try to stop the bleeding that was restricting his heart. His chest was opened, but he could not be saved. The lead physician called the time of death, and everyone but the techs left the room. We could hear the sobs of his parents. It was almost surreal.

As we quickly cleaned the blood from the floor and cleaned and draped John's body so that his parents would be able to see him, the silence in the room was deafening. Once we were finished and allowed the parents into the room, the crying became intense and my heart was aching.

A fifteen-year-old boy is not supposed to die like that, I thought. I couldn't reconcile this tragedy, initially. Instead of holding in my feelings, I grabbed one of the nurses and expressed my feelings. **I began to cry and thought that I may not be cut out for this line of work. She explained to me that it is human to cry, and that not all patients are going to live despite our best efforts. All we can do is give it our best effort. We are not God.**

Although I still think about John to this very day, I learned that we cannot save everyone, and that death is a part of life. All we can do is try our best, and perhaps it's up to a Higher Power to decide if the patient lives or dies.

QUALITIES
▶ Humility
▶ Empathy
▶ Ability to work under pressure

DO...
✓ Stay cool under pressure and do the best you can without involving emotion.
✓ Stay focused on the job at hand.
✓ Express your feelings to someone.
✓ Understand that life is fragile and fleeting

DON'T...
✗ Don't panic
✗ Don't let your emotions get in the way of your job.
✗ Don't keep your feelings bottled up inside.
✗ Don't beat yourself up for not being able to save every patient.

If we remember one thing about you, what should that be?

This question should be very easy to answer. I've spent a lot of time talking about the importance of pointing out your Qualities to the committee. Since they want you to mention "one thing," and you can't list all of them, keep your answer simple and brief.

EXAMPLE ANSWER
I would like the committee to remember that **I am a team player**.

QUALITY

▶ Team player

DO...

✓ Mention only one quality.

✓ Follow instructions. Only mention *one* thing you want them to remember about you.

DON'T...

✗ Don't mention multiple qualities.

✗ Don't be unprepared for this question. What *do* you want the committee to remember about you?

How do physician assistants fit into the healthcare model?

This question is asked to see if you understand where PAs fit into the healthcare team. Be careful not to describe a hierarchy; don't say that PAs are "above" nurses on the healthcare team, or "below" physicians.

EXAMPLE ANSWER

The best way to answer this question is to discuss my experiences working with PAs on a medical floor in a community hospital. I worked as a CNA, so I got to see first-hand how the entire healthcare team worked together with a common goal of caring for the patient.

For instance, the PAs working on our floor were all hospitalists. Although they were the primary care provider for their assigned patients admitted to the unit, **they had to work collaboratively with many team members to coordinate the care of the patient**. The patient always came first. The PA had to provide updates to the patient's primary care physician and work with every team member involved in the patient's care, including consulting physicians, nurse practitioners, CNAs, allied health professionals, family members, clergy, and so on. The PA working as a hospitalist may be the patient's primary care provider in the hospital, however, the collaboration and coordination with the other caregivers was an essential component of treating the patient.

There is no hierarchy when it comes to patient care. I like to use the analogy of the PA being one spoke on a wheel of the healthcare team. If everyone on the team does an effective job of caring for the patient, meaning if all the spokes on the wheel are the same length, the wheel runs very smoothly. However, if any participant on the team falls short, the spokes become uneven, and the wheel will become ineffective. The PAs job is to keep her ego out of the job, and to keep her spoke "right-sized." Teamwork is the key to success.

QUALITIES
▶ Experience working with PAs and other healthcare professionals
▶ Collaboration
▶ Team player

DO...
✓ Stress the collaborative nature of the PA profession.
✓ Put the patient at the center of care.
✓ Stress the words "healthcare team."
✓ Give an example using your own experiences working in healthcare, or your observations from shadowing.

DON'T...
✗ Don't mention a hierarchy.
✗ Don't focus exclusively on the PAs role.
✗ Don't downplay the role of *any* providers on the healthcare team.

How do you see the healthcare system changing in the next ten years, and how will it affect PAs?

At present, nobody can predict what the healthcare system is going to look like under President Trump. What we do know is that there will be more patients entering the healthcare system, and there is a projected shortage of physicians into the next decade. This situation will provide a gap between healthcare providers available to treat the new patients entering the system, and PAs are perfectly positioned to fill that gap.

EXAMPLE ANSWER

The healthcare system in this country is in constant flux. Healthcare has also become a political hotbed of discussion. The Affordable Care Act provided access to care for many patients who may not have had access before, resulting in an influx of new patients into the healthcare system.

Keep in mind that the Affordable Care Act will likely change significantly or be abolished soon.

In any case, the fact is that there will be an influx of new patients into the healthcare system, and **there is a projected physician shortage of 120,000 by the year 2030. PAs are perfectly positioned to fill this gap**.

QUALITY
▶ Understanding the future role of PAs in healthcare

DO...
✓ Study the role of the PA in healthcare.
✓ Speak with physicians and PAs about their feelings on the future of healthcare.
✓ Paint a positive picture for PAs in the future.
✓ Stay current with healthcare reform.
✓ Use specific examples from journals or articles to make your case.

DON'T...

✘ Don't forget to do your homework on this topic.

✘ Don't say that healthcare reform will be positive for PAs, and not back up your answer with examples and facts.

I see you have a few W's on your transcript during your freshman year, can you explain why that is?

Okay, so you didn't have the best year when you were a freshman. Hopefully your grades trended upward in subsequent years. You are not alone. The key here is not to make excuses. Take responsibility for the withdrawals and be honest as to why you felt the need to do so. The committee is looking for honesty, and a reasonable explanation.

Remember, if you received an interview, you have what it takes to become a PA student. Briefly explain the situation and move on.

EXAMPLE ANSWER

I take full responsibility for the W's on my transcript. **I initially had a tough time transitioning from high school to college**, but as you will also see on my transcripts **my trend was upward since my freshman year**.

QUALITIES

▶ Accepting responsibility

▶ Honesty

▶ Maturity

DO...

✓ Accept responsibility.

✓ Be honest.

✓ Point out how you improved your grades the next three years.

✓ Anticipate this question.

DON'T...

✘ Don't make excuses!

✘ Don't give a long, drawn out answer. Keep it brief and move on.

If you could change one thing about the PA profession, what would it be?

To be able to intelligently answer this question, you will need to speak with many PAs and do your homework. The AAPA website is a great place to start. Frequent the site and read about the hot topics relative to the PA profession. Be sure you understand the basics of any issues you uncover and be willing to take a stance. The example answer will cover one such topic that is currently in the news and will affect all PAs if enacted. You can read about this issue on the AAPA website and Google the topic to gain a good understanding of the issue.

EXAMPLE ANSWER

The PA profession has been growing since its inception fifty years ago. I believe any changes made to the profession would need to benefit patients and the PA profession itself.

While doing my research, I've found that there are two current issues of concern: PAs: changing their name from physician assistant to physician associate, and the position on "Full Practice Authority and Responsibility" (FPAR).

I've considered both issues carefully, and I don't think I would vote "yes" on the name change unless PAs are granted Full Practice Authority and Responsibility. However, I do support the AAPA's FPAR stance on full practice authority. From what I've read, and from speaking with many practicing physician assistants, nurse practitioners are preferred in many clinical settings over PAs because NPs are independent practitioners (in many states), and because they do not require as much oversight. In fact, the VA healthcare system has already granted nurse practitioners Full Practice Authority and Responsibility.

If PAs are going to compete with nurse practitioners in the job market, I think the FPAR proposal, if enacted, will be a positive change for PAs and for patients. With the increased gap between health care providers and patients, coupled with the projected physician shortage over the next several years, when FPAR is enacted, PAs will lose fewer jobs to nurse practitioners in the future.

The AAPA's Joint Task Force on the future of PA practice authority recommends adopting policy to do four things:

1. Continue to emphasize a commitment to team-based practice.
2. Eliminate laws that require PAs to report a supervising physician in order to practice.
3. Establish autonomous state boards, with voting member- ship comprised mostly of PAs, to license, regulate, and discipline PAs.
4. Ensure PAs are eligible to be reimbursed directly by public and private insurance.

I agree with the Task Force recommendation, and I would vote "yes" if I were polled.

QUALITIES

▶ Experienced with issues facing the PA profession
▶ Reasoning skills
▶ Decisive
▶ Researched on profession
▶ Knows the issues

DO...

✓ Visit the AAPA website to find out about the most current topics involving the PA profession.
✓ Develop a thorough understanding of these topics.
✓ Formulate your own opinion on the topic.
✓ Google the topic and read about the various viewpoints from practicing PAs.

✓ Speak with as many PAs as you can and ask what they might change relative to the profession.
✓ Keep current with the status of FPAR for the PA profession.

DON'T...

✗ Don't say, "I wouldn't change anything."
✗ Don't forget to thoroughly research the topic and be able to explain your reasoning to the committee.
✗ Don't get caught off-guard!

Do you think PAs should be called Physician Assistants or Physician Associates? Explain your answer.

This question has been a topic of debate since I became a PA in 1994. In the mid-sixties, PAs were initially called Physician Associates. However, due some pushback from physicians having concerns with the implication of the name "physician associate," the profession changed the name to physician assistant.

There really is no right or wrong answer to this question, if you can intelligently defend your answer. As this is a common interview question, think about it beforehand and weigh the pros and cons of your answer.

From what I've learned working with PA school applicants, most applicants automatically answer, "I would change the name to physician associate." I think they believe this is the answer that the interviewer wants to hear. I also think (my opinion only) that there is a lot of ego involved. I follow this debate on the PA Forum (physicianassistantforum.com), and many respondents simply say, "I'm nobody's assistant!"

I know many PAs will disagree with my philosophy, but I rarely here an articulate response as to why we should change the name after fifty-years.

EXAMPLE ANSWER

I would choose to keep the name of the profession to physician assistant. After more than fifty-years, the profession continues to grow, and is consistently ranked by the Bureau of Labor Statistics as one of the top career fields in the country. Patient satisfaction with PAs is also ranked extremely high; right up there with physicians and nurse practitioners.

I'm not sure that making a name change at this point would improve upon the success of the profession. Most patients know what a PA is, and what a PA does. Changing the name would also require a period of time to reeducate patients and may cause confusion.

I've also considered the logistics of a name change. I would imagine that changing the name on all the literature from the AAPA, state chapters of the AAPA, PA schools, websites, and other brochures and printed materials, would cost a great deal of money.

Although I believe the name "physician associate" better describes the duties of a PA, I'm a big believer that "if it's not broken, don't fix it." If PAs are granted Full Practice Authority and Responsibility, then I might reconsider my decision.

QUALITIES
▶ Decisive
▶ Thinking outside of the box
▶ Thoughtful
▶ Leadership

DO...
✓ Think about the question and come up with your *own* answer and reasons for choosing that answer. If you go online, you'll discover that many PAs favor the name change. In my opinion, there is a bit of ego involved in that decision.
✓ Think outside of the box.
✓ Read discussions on both sides of the issue and take a stand.

DON'T...

- ✘ Don't forget that you will need to justify your answer.
- ✘ Try not to sound too clichéd when answering this question.
- ✘ Don't go along with the rest of the herd because you think you should play it safe.

Who inspired you the most in life, and why?

EXAMPLE ANSWER

I would say my grandmother. She taught me that just about **anything is achievable through hard work, dedication, and courage**. She had five children, and then she and my grandfather fostered (and adopted) three more. As the kids got into their teens, she decided she wanted to do more with her life. My grandmother applied for and got into nursing school. This was in the Midwest in the late 1960s, so it was somewhat shocking that a married mother would go back to school. At first, she was afraid that she wouldn't be able to measure up. But, **she stuck to her guns, studied hard, graduated, and got a job**. All that time, she still guided her kids all through their own education.

QUALITIES

- ▶ Persistence
- ▶ Dealing with fears in life

DO...

- ✓ Explain *why* that person inspired you.
- ✓ Be sure to discuss the lesson you learned.
- ✓ Think hard about this question, and try to remember a lesson that you still use/remember today, and how that lesson would relate to the Qualities of being a PA student/PA.

DON'T...

- ✘ Don't say, "I can't think of any one person."
- ✘ Don't say, "Many people inspired me in life."

What can you tell us about the history of the PA profession?

If you plan on convincing the admissions committee that you are passionate and motivated to become a PA, you better research the profession and learn about its history. There is a lot of information about the history of the PA profession on the Internet. There is no excuse for not being well-informed on this topic. Neglect to do your homework at your own peril.

EXAMPLE ANSWER

In the mid-1960s, navy hospital corpsman returned from Vietnam with a considerable amount of medical training and experience, but no place in the civilian world to capitalize on that experience. At the same time, the country was experiencing a shortage of primary care physicians, especially in rural and underserved areas. Dr. Eugene Stead, of the Duke University Medical School, came up with a solution to this problem. **Dr. Stead, who is considered the founder of the PA profession, assembled the first class of physician assistants in 1965 comprised of former navy corpsman. The PA curriculum was based on the fast-track training of physicians during World War II.**

From those first few navy corpsmen who graduated from Duke on October 6th, 1967, there are currently 250 PA programs in the United States and 123,000 PAs as of 2018.

QUALITIES
▶ Knowledge of the history of the PA profession
▶ Passion for the PA profession

DO...
✓ Know the history of the PA profession.
✓ Visit the Physician Assistant History Society at https://pahx.org/oral-histories/

DON'T...

✘ Don't neglect to research this topic.

✘ Don't respond, "I don't know much about the history of the PA profession."

What was the last book you read?

Although you can expect to be asked about your qualities and medical experience at your PA school interview, you should also be prepared to be asked personal questions like, "What was the last book you read?" The interviewer wants to get a feel for what kind of person you are when you are not working or studying. If you are struggling to answer this question now, be sure to read something before your interview.

I know that many of you are heavily involved in school and working and it may be difficult to have a lot of leisure time to read. However, try to set aside some time to read a book that reinforces the same Qualities that you bring to the table as a PA school applicant. Remember to be honest, and name a book that you've actually read. The last thing you want to happen is give an answer about a book that you have not read when one of the committee members has, and begins asking you questions about it. You will lose total credibility doing this. Also, be careful about naming controversial books, especially those on political topics.

EXAMPLE ANSWER

The last book I read was, "Think and Grow Rich" by Napoleon Hill. This self-help classic is not just centered on making money and becoming rich. This book teaches **valuable lessons on goal setting, persistence, accomplishing your personal goals by helping others achieve their goals, and drives home the point that; What the mind of man can conceive and believe, it can achieve**.

I would imagine that Dr. Eugene Stead, founder of the PA profession, utilized many of these principles to start the PA profession.

QUALITIES

▶ Goal oriented
▶ Persistence
▶ Having belief in oneself

DO...

✓ Focus on a piece of work that reflects positively on your qualities.
✓ Emphasize why you chose to read that title.
✓ Read a book before your interview, if you haven't read a book in a while!

DON'T...

✗ Don't focus on dark or negative books.
✗ Don't focus on political books.
✗ Don't mention a book you haven't read. The interviewer may have read the book you mentioned and ask you questions about the plot, or anything else of importance to him.

What do you value most in a classmate or coworker?

This question is really a reflection about your own values. The committee wants to see what's important to you as a coworker or classmate.

EXAMPLE ANSWER

I really value teammates who are supportive, dedicated to the job, and willing to go the extra mile to accomplish the task at hand. I worked as a technician in an emergency room and we would often be short-handed on busy nights. The staff often stayed late, well after our shift was over, **to help with the patient flow until the physicians, nurses, and technicians were caught up with patients.**

QUALITIES

▶ Supportive
▶ Dedicated
▶ Willing to go the extra mile
▶ Team player

DO...

✓ Choose qualities that would make a good classmate or coworker and infuse them into your answer.
✓ Use an anecdote to demonstrate the qualities you value.
✓ I strongly recommend that you infuse "team player" as a quality.

DON'T...

✗ Don't say, "Someone who likes to party like I do after work."
✗ Don't mention qualities that are not relevant to being a good classmate or PA.

Name a time when you were dependent on others.

I hope you know by now that the PA profession, by definition, is a dependent profession. The interviewer is looking to see if you truly understand the nature of being a dependent practitioner, and how you may have been in a dependent role in the past. (Be mindful that if FPAR is implemented for PAs, the profession will no longer be a dependent one.)

EXAMPLE ANSWER

As a former navy corpsman and air force officer, I spent seven years in the military. From day one, we were trained to **work as a team and look out for one another. We learned the importance of following a chain of command**. When given a "lawful" order by our supervisors, we followed the order to conclusion, and **learned to develop trust and humility**. I believe both traits are relevant to the physician-PA relationship.

QUALITIES

▶ Teamwork
▶ Supporting teammates
▶ Following orders of superiors
▶ Trust
▶ Humility

DO...

✓ Mention qualities that match those you'll need as a PA student and as a PA.
✓ Think about this question before your interview.

DON'T...

✘ Don't say, "I've always been very independent."
✘ Don't look at being dependent as a weakness.

How would you describe your personality?

This may seem like an innocuous question, but I assure you if you answer too hastily you may end up sounding like a "vanilla" applicant. Remember, your goal is to become the Perfect Applicant.

Interviewers ask this question to see if you can think on your feet, be creative, and separate yourself from the other applicants.

EXAMPLE ANSWER

I would describe my personality in three ways: **I am energized by challenges and problems, I'm a team player and I do whatever it takes to get the job done, and I can hit the ground running and come up to speed faster than anyone I know.**

QUALITIES

▶ Welcomes challenges
▶ Hard worker
▶ Fast learner

DO...

✓ Show the committee what makes you unique.
✓ Convince the committee that you have the qualities they're looking for in a Perfect Applicant.
✓ Be specific with your answers.
✓ Ask your friends for input, and make a list of personality traits that best describe you.

DON'T...

✗ Don't give "vanilla" answers, "I'm a hard worker." This answer shows no imagination.
✗ Don't sound like every other applicant.
✗ Don't forget to take an *honest* inventory of yourself.

What preparation have you made to become a PA?

This is an important question. You'll need to show passion and humility, but not come off as arrogant. This is a question where you can really separate yourself from the competition. Here you want to take the ADCOM through your action plan. You will just need to highlight some of the areas that are most important. Show your interviewer that you have been pursuing your dream of becoming a PA with diligence and persistence.

EXAMPLE ANSWER

I understand that the PA profession is physically, mentally, and spiritually challenging. Therefore, I have diligently prepared myself in each of these areas.

I exercise daily to improve my stamina. I understand as a PA student I will be working long hours, both in the classroom and on clinical rotations. Exercising is a fantastic way to stay energized and relieve stress.

I joined the American Academy of Physician Assistants (AAPA) to keep current on issues facing PAs at the national level. I also joined the Connecticut Academy of Physician Assistants (ConnAPA) to keep current with issues relative to PAs at the state level. I've shadowed several PAs and asked a lot of questions about the profession at the clinical level. I also frequent the PA Forum and threads from current PAs and Pre-PAs.

(Note: More than half of the PA school applicants that I speak with in my mock Interview sessions do not know that the AAPA and state chapters, constituent chapters of the AAPA, even exist!)

Finally, I've been reading books on mindfulness. **I've been practicing techniques to help me stay "in the moment" and "be present," which will go a long way to keep me focused during PA school, and when I become a PA.**

QUALITIES
▶ Understanding of the PA profession
▶ Joining the AAPA and ConnAPA; staying involved in issues facing PAs at the national and state level
▶ Learning how to maintain focus

DO...
✓ Join the AAPA and your state chapter of the AAPA.
✓ Frequent the websites of the above organizations.
✓ Learn about current issues facing the PA profession.
✓ Frequent the website of the state chapter where you'll be interviewing.

DON'T...
✘ Don't try to "wing it" when it comes to your answer.
✘ Don't ignore the physical and spiritual components of this question.

What does it mean to be a dependent practitioner?

The interviewer will want to make sure that you understand the dependent nature of the PA profession. This question does not ask you to explain the entire role of a PA. If the interviewer wants you to expand on your answer, be prepared to talk about autonomy, etc.

EXAMPLE ANSWER

By definition, PAs are dependent practitioners, PAs must always work under the license of a supervising physician.

QUALITY

▶ Understanding the dependent nature of the profession

DO...

✓ Provide a *brief* answer to the question being asked; keep it simple.

✓ Be able to expand your answer *if* you're challenged about working autonomously, etc.

DON'T...

✗ Don't read too much into this question. The answer consists of one sentence.

✗ Don't tell your interviewer that your supervising physician will dictate *all* of your daily decisions.

Why are you a good fit for the PA profession?

This question provides the opportunity to list all the qualities you possess to become a great PA student, and ultimately a great PA. Here is where you can summarize your qualities into a brief, concise manner in the form of a laundry list. Review your CASPA application and essay and develop a list of your key qualities. Use hard numbers and facts, where necessary, to demonstrate these qualities. Your answer to this question will also provide you with an opportunity to tell the committee about all of your wonderful Qualities; especially if the interview is a closed one (the committee doesn't have access to your CASPA application.)

EXAMPLE ANSWER

I believe I am a good fit for the PA profession because I have **demonstrated the passion and motivation to become a PA. I have 4500 hours of hands-on medical experience working as an EMT, Medical Assistant, and emergency room technician. I have a 3.7 GPA and above average GRE scores**, so I know that if I'm selected to this program, I have the academic ability to complete the program and pass the PANCE exam.

I am a **team player**. **I was captain of my Division I college soccer team**, and as an EMT and ER tech **I've had to work in collaboration with multiple medical disciplines under stressful situations.** I am a **lifelong learner**. I am 8 credits shy of completing my master's degree. **I am also a compassionate and empathetic person.** During my 4,500 hours of medical experience, I learned how to **communicate** with my patients, ease their fears, and show a genuine concern for their wellbeing.

I believe I have many more qualities that would make me a good fit for the PA profession, but the qualities I just mentioned are my greatest strengths.

QUALITIES
▶ Passion and motivation
▶ Extensive medical experience
▶ Academic ability
▶ Collaboration
▶ Lifelong learner
▶ Empathy
▶ Communication skills

DO...

✓ Write down a list of your Qualities and be sure to mention them throughout the interview, and especially when answering this question.

✓ Spend a lot of time reviewing your experiences in life and uncover as many Qualities as you can.

✓ Be prepared to list these Qualities in a brief and concise manner.

DON'T...

✗ Don't make up Qualities that you can't back up or demonstrate.

✗ Don't be unprepared for this question. You can't "wing it."

✗ Don't forget about "transferable skills" (from a non-medical job).

What will you do if you do not get accepted to PA school this year?

This question is one that can be a little intimidating. Many applicants feel as though they may not get accepted when asked this question. Don't concern yourself. This question is very common, asked of all applicants, and is not personal to you. The committee simply wants to know if you'll give up on your dream of becoming a PA, or if you'll continue to improve your application and apply again next year.

EXAMPLE ANSWER

The first thing that I'll do if I don't get accepted to PA school this year will be to **contact the PA programs where I've interviewed/ applied and see if I can find out specifics of where I fell short. I will take that advice and continue to improve my application before the next cycle and apply again next year**.

QUALITIES

▶ Persistent

▶ Motivated

DO...

✓ Show that you are not a quitter and that you are still motivated to become a PA.

✓ Call each program that you may have been rejected from and try to speak with someone who can give you *specific* reasons why you were not chosen to interview, or if you did interview, why you weren't accepted.

✓ Keep a positive attitude. Remember, "Quitters never win, and winners never quit."

DON'T...

✗ Don't be intimidated by this question; it's not personal.

✗ Don't complain or pester the program trying to find out why you were not accepted; attempt one call, then leave it be.

✗ Don't be surprised if the program gives you the generic answer; "We have a large applicant pool, and we can only take fifty people; it's very competitive..."

Do you have any questions for us?

Typically, at the end of every interview session, the committee will ask if you have any questions. Please don't say, "no." This is your opportunity to find out the qualities and values the program is looking for in applicants they accept to their program. Once you know the qualities, you can infuse them into your answers. That is why I stress attending the Open House if possible. At the Open House, you will have many opportunities to speak with students and faculty, and you can ask about the qualities the program values the most.

EXAMPLE ANSWER

Yes, thank you. I have three questions that I would like to ask:

1. What are the three most important qualities you look for in a competitive applicant?

2. What type of applicants are most successful in this program?
3. If you could describe the culture of this program in three words, what would they be?

QUALITIES
▶ Motivation
▶ Inquisitive
▶ Not afraid to challenge the committee

DO...
✓ Ask questions!
✓ Use these questions to learn about the qualities the program values.
✓ Remember that you are a consumer. You will likely invest over $100,000 of your hard-earned money and two years of your life at this institution. Let them sell *you* on why you should attend their program.
✓ Prepare your questions ahead of time.

DON'T...
✖ Don't say, "No thank you, you've answered all of my questions."
✖ Don't become intimidated.
✖ Don't ask questions that you should already know the answers to. For instance, if the program's mission statement is published on their website, don't ask them "What is the mission of this program?"

On the next page, I've provided you with a Perfect Applicant blueprint. Feel free to make copies and practice coming up with your own Perfect Applicant answers.

PERFECT APPLICANT ANSWERS

Copy and fill out this preparation sheet for each of your PA school interviews. Following this format will help you focus on your qualities and prepare answers for the most commonly asked questions.

Question: "Tell me about yourself..."

Qualities	**Multipliers**
_____	_____
_____	_____
_____	_____
_____	_____

Success Story

_____

_____

_____

_____

Perfect Applicant Answer

_____

_____

_____

_____

_____

_____

_____

_____

_____

_____

_____

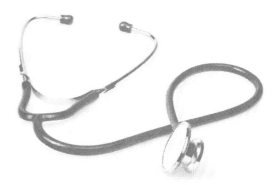

CHAPTER 3

Behavioral Questions

In today's competitive PA school interview process, Behavioral Questions are responsible for more rejection letters than any other type of questions. In this chapter, I'm going to show you a simple trick for answering any behavioral question with ease. This will prevent you from failing the interview due to lack of knowledge in dealing with these difficult questions; especially since they are becoming more popular with admissions committees.

There are many possibilities for how an interview can go wrong, but the fact is none are more brutal and unpredictable than behavioral interview questions. Furthermore, it has been my experience, through conducting hundreds of mock interviews with PA school applicants, that more and more applicants are totally clueless when it comes to answering behavioral interview questions. In fact, many applicants who work with me after reapplying report that their inability to answer behavioral questions was one of the most embarrassing things to happen to them in their past interviews.

Think about it: How would you feel sitting in the hot seat with the interviewer staring at you right across the table, and you have nothing to say? You're not exactly going to come across as the Perfect Applicant! And the fact of the matter is, you cannot avoid behavioral questions. Why? Because more PA programs are utilizing them to weed out weaker applicants, and you don't want that to be you!

Many PA programs now use behavioral questions as their preferred way to determine their top candidates. Behavioral questions allow the interviewer to uncover the specific skills, knowledge, and experience you have.

Here is a simple analogy. If you ever watched any of the many crime shows on television, you'll notice that a murder suspect moves up higher on the list if he or she has a history of violent criminal activity in the past. His past record is a strong indicator of his current behavior.

Behavioral questions are meant to ask you about your previous behavior or actions, that will indicate how you'll react in the future as a PA.

While a traditional interview includes straightforward questions like, "How do you handle stress?" the same behavioral question would be, "Tell us about a time when you had to handle a stressful situation, and how you dealt with it." The traditional form of this question is very simple to answer; I exercise/meditate/do Yoga, etc. The behavioral question is much more difficult and requires an example of a *specific* situation or task.

Behavioral interview questions can be immediately recognized by the wording used. Here are some examples of how a typical behavioral question may start:

- ► Tell me about a time...
- ► Can you give me an example of...?
- ► What was the biggest/most important/most difficult...?
- ► Describe a time when...

As soon as the interviewer begins a question in this fashion, you should immediately recognize that a behavioral question is coming your way. You will need to provide an appropriate story that highlights the different competencies and skillsets the program is looking for. The problem is that most applicants might have a general idea of how to answer these questions, but the answers usually come out way too long and unfocused and won't portray the applicant in the best light.

That's why you need to be aware of the behavioral questions you are likely to be asked, and then create stories or scenarios that are adapted to the relevant competencies of a PA.

Here is a list of common behavioral-based interview questions:

1. **Teamwork Interview Questions.** If the situation calls for an example of being a team player, you should provide an example that demonstrates how you work well with others.

2. **Leadership Interview Questions.** If people may be reporting to you, or you've had to take charge of a difficult situation at a job, you will be expected to answer questions about your ability to lead and motivate others.

3. **Handling Conflict Interview Questions.** The PA profession requires a lot of interaction with patients and multiple health-care providers (or challenging situations with other colleagues). The interviewer may ask you for examples of how you handled or defused tricky situations.

4. **Problem Solving.** Being a PA requires critical thinking skills, and the admissions committee may want to know about challenging issues/situations that required some innovation or outside-the-box thinking.

5. **Biggest Failure Interview Questions.** More and more PA school interviewers are asking failure questions. Whether you like it or not, you need to be prepared to have a satisfactory answer. Be sure to mention what you learned from this failure.

For many of you who are recent graduates, and really have not hit the workforce yet, you may have a little more difficulty answering behavioral questions. Keep in mind that behavioral questions don't have to be related to healthcare or a past job. You may need to relate stories from your education, team sports, or volunteer positions. The key is to relate your answer to the Qualities being sought in the question.

Here are six rules for answering behavioral questions:

1. Your answer/example must be specific.
2. Your examples should be concise.
3. Your examples should include the action you took.
4. Your examples must demonstrate your role.
5. Your examples should be relevant to the question asked.
6. Your stories must have a result.

Preparing for Behavioral Interviews

PA programs have a defined set of skills and key competencies they desire in a strong applicant. These skillsets and competencies could include: decision making and problem solving, leadership, motivation, communication, interpersonal skills, critical thinking skills, the ability to work within a team, compassion, the ability to work autonomously, and the ability to influence others. In preparation for your PA school interview, research your answers to the following questions:

1. What are the necessary skills and key competencies programs desire in PA students?
2. What skills are necessary to be a physician assistant student?
3. What makes a successful PA school applicant?
4. What would make a PA school applicant unsuccessful?
5. What is the most challenging part of being a PA?

The STAR Technique

A fantastic way to answer behavioral questions is to use the **STAR** technique. STAR is an acronym for: The **S**ituation or **T**ask, the **A**ction you took, and the **R**esult (or outcome) of the action.

For example, you may need to recall a time when you had to work under stressful conditions (situation or task). To handle the situation, you had to organize your employees/classmates/coworkers and discuss options to achieve a goal (action). Following the plan you developed, you were able to accomplish the goal on time (result). Using the STAR technique is a powerful way for you to frame your experiences.

Here are few tips for answering behavioral questions:

- Don't ramble and go off on a tangent.
- Listen carefully to the question.
- Practice answering behavioral questions before your interview.
- Pause before you answer; don't feel the need to rush your answer, especially with behavioral questions.

The following chart will help you understand the STAR technique format:

Situation or **T**ask	Describe the situation you were in or the task you were assigned. You must describe a specific event or situation, not a generalized description of what you have done in the past. Be sure to give enough detail for the interviewer to understand the scenario. The situation can be an event from a previous job or from a volunteer experience that is relevant to the question.
Action	Describe the action you took, and be sure to keep the focus on yourself. Even if you are discussing a group project or effort, describe what you did—not the efforts of the team. Don't tell what you might have done. Tell what you did.
Result	What happened because of your action? How did the situation/task end? What did you accomplish? What did you learn?

Use examples from internships, classes, school projects, activities, team participation, community service, hobbies, and work experience as examples of your past behavior. In addition, feel free to use examples of special accomplishments, whether professional or personal, such as scoring a winning touchdown in the championship game, being elected to office in an organization, winning a prize for your artwork, surfing a big wave, or raising money for charity.

Wherever possible, quantify your results. Numbers always impress committee members.

Remember that many behavioral questions try to uncover how you responded to negative situations. You'll need to have examples of negative experiences ready but try to choose negative experiences that you've made the best of, or better yet, those that had positive outcomes.

Here's an effective way to prepare for behavioral-based interview questions:

- ▸ Identify six to eight examples from your past experiences where you demonstrated behaviors and skills that PA school admissions committees seek.
- ▸ Half of your examples should be totally positive, like accomplishments or meeting goals.
- ▸ The other half should be situations that may have started out negatively, but either ended positively or where you made the best of this outcome.
- ▸ Vary your examples. If you are a college student, examples from high school may be irrelevant. Try to use examples from the past year.
- ▸ Use the STAR technique to answer these questions.

The night before your interview is not the time to prepare for behavioral questions. You should start preparing for them long before your interview.

In the interview, listen carefully to each question, identify the question as a behavioral question (Tell us about a time when...), recall a situation that you reviewed before the interview that pertains the question being asked, and immediately think "STAR" technique.

Sample Behavioral Interview Questions

▸ Tell me about a time you worked effectively under pressure.

▸ Tell me about a stressful situation you experienced in college and how you handled it.

▸ Tell me about a time you made a mistake and had to tell your boss or professor.

▸ Tell me how you would you deal with a coworker who wasn't doing his share of the work.

▸ Tell me about a time that you had a conflict with a team member and how you handled it.

▸ Tell me about a time when you were disappointed in your performance.

▸ Tell me about a time you had to build a relationship with someone you didn't like.

▸ Tell me about a difficult decision you've made in the last year.

▸ Tell me about a time when you tried to accomplish something and failed.

BEHAVIORAL INTERVIEW QUESTIONS

Tell me/us about a time when you had to overcome obstacles to get a job done.

The interview committee wants to know if you can think for yourself, and if you are a problem solver.

EXAMPLE ANSWER

SITUATION: While in college, **I was involved in a group assignment where four of us had to do research on the Hepatitis C virus and prepare a presentation on our findings to faculty members and students in the science department.** I was assigned to this group late in the process. During my first meeting with the group, I quickly realized that although a large portion of the research they gathered was very thorough, it was not very useful for a presentation. The information was way too technical, and not very conducive to a slideshow presentation for our target audience.

ACTION: **Rather than suggesting the group start over from scratch, I took the initiative to restructure the complex information into a simpler format.** Everyone agreed with the changes and we incorporated the data into an effective and targeted presentation.

RESULT: **Our group received an award for the presentation. I take immense pride in being able to come up with simple, effective solutions to seemingly impossible problems.**

QUALITY
▶ Problem-solver
▶ Initiative

DO...
✓ Take a moment to brag a bit. This is a time to show off your problem-solving skills, but don't go overboard.
✓ The applicant took what could have been a disastrous research project and turned it into an award-winning presentation. Rather than starting over from scratch, she looked at the data already collected and revised it into a much simpler format that the audience would be able to digest and understand.
✓ This answer lets the interviewer know that she can think outside of the box and is a creative problem solver.

DON'T...
✗ Don't worry about telling a story where you solved all the world's problems.
✗ Don't exaggerate your accomplishment.
✗ Don't take credit for something you didn't do.

Tell me about a time when you had to handle a stressful situation.

You can count on being asked this question. The interviewer is looking for a specific example of a stressful situation you've had to face and how you resolved it. He may also want to see what you consider to be stressful.

EXAMPLE ANSWER

SITUATION: **I started a new job as a medical assistant in a family practice. After working there for a week, I noticed that the medical providers were complaining a lot about the examination rooms not being stocked appropriately with supplies.** A provider would come out in the middle of an office visit and become angry that there were no paper towels, no band aids, no gauze, etc. We all felt like we were walking on eggshells. The office manager held a meeting and came down heavy on all of us. I felt as though my job might be in jeopardy, and I had only been there for a week.

ACTION: I also have a lot of experience as a medical assistant, so I suggested that the MAs all get together to discuss the problem. **I proposed that we come up with a checklist and place it outside the door of every treatment room.** Every morning, we would all be responsible to complete the checklist and stock the rooms appropriately.

RESULT: This system worked, and the providers were very appreciative. **I was complimented by the office manager for coming up with the solution and for alleviating a constant source of stress in the practice.**

QUALITIES

▶ Ability to handle stress
▶ Innovative
▶ Problem-solver
▶ Leadership

DO...

✓ Use a specific and real example of a stressful situation.
✓ State the problem.
✓ Describe exactly what you did to solve the problem.
✓ Make yourself the hero without going overboard.

DON'T...

✗ Don't ramble; keep it succinct and related to the problem.
✗ Don't exaggerate.

Tell me about a time when you had to adapt quickly to a change.

There is one constant in this world—change! The admissions committee wants to know that you will able to adapt to any given situation in PA school, and, more importantly, as a practicing PA.

EXAMPLE ANSWER

SITUATION: I was working as a phlebotomist in a primary care clinic. We were in the middle of a flu epidemic and three of our medical assistants called out sick. **I was cross-trained as a medical assistant and I decided to wear two hats that day, performing both medical assistant duties as well as my phlebotomy duties.**

ACTION: **To keep the flow moving in the clinic and not fall behind with my lab duties, I had the front office staff call my lab patients and reschedule them for my lunch hour. I continued my medical assistant duties while fitting in blood draws when I could during the rest of the day and at lunch.**

RESULT: **At the end of the day, we did not have one patient walk out, and I accomplished all my phlebotomy duties. The physician who owned the practice stopped in the lab before I left for the day and thanked me for doing "an excellent job." He offered me a half-day off because of my efforts.**

QUALITIES

- ▶ Adaptability
- ▶ Problem solver
- ▶ Team player
- ▶ Innovative

DO...

- ✓ Show that you took charge of a stressful situation and solved a problem.
- ✓ Show that you have personal initiative.
- ✓ Express that you are a team player.
- ✓ Indicate that you are willing to sacrifice some of your own time and comfort to get the job done.

DON'T...

- ✗ Don't exaggerate.
- ✗ Don't make up a situation that never happened.

Tell me about a time someone on your team didn't do his or her job, and how you resolved the problem.

Being on a healthcare team requires that everyone on that team operates smoothly and collaboratively. If you have one employee who is having difficulty or not doing their part, it can throw off the entire team, and ultimately impact patient care. Admissions committees feel that they are the gatekeepers for the PA profession, as well as their particular programs. The committee wants to know that the applicants they select have basic leadership qualities, which means being a problem-solver.

EXAMPLE ANSWER

SITUATION: **In my last position as a supervisor**, I was responsible for several other individuals, one of whom seemed to always be a step behind the rest of the team and consistently missed deadlines.

ACTION: **I took him aside and I discovered, through the course of our discussion, that he had been promoted from another department but never given the necessary training for his new position.** He was terrified to ask for help because he thought that if it became known that he lacked this training, he would be immediately fired. Instead, he had been struggling and essentially learning on his own.

RESULT: Rather than having him fired, **I realized what he needed was a little help.** We worked out a schedule where we could meet up and I could mentor him. By working together and helping him go over the materials and learn his job, I could retain a valuable employee. Now, rather than slowing down the team, he became an integral member of it.

QUALITIES
▶ Empathy
▶ Mentorship

DO...
✓ Show that you can take the time to listen to a coworker who may be struggling.
✓ Provide examples of your ability to successfully lead your team, including supporting members who may be struggling.

DON'T...
✘ Don't brag about deceitful techniques you have employed in the past.
✘ Don't assume you know what the problem is, then act on that assumption.

Tell me about a time when your communication skills made a difference.

Being an effective communicator is a necessary quality if you are going to be a healthcare provider. Obviously, PAs communicate with patients every day, sometimes to explain treatment regimens or diagnosis, and sometimes to persuade patients about why they need to lose weight to treat their high blood pressure or diabetes. Effective communicators make better providers.

EXAMPLE ANSWER

SITUATION: One project I worked on in college involved developing a curriculum for a program dealing with cultural similarities in everyday life. **The challenge was to communicate with my team members and get them as excited about their roles in the project as I was about mine.**

ACTION: **I met with each member of the team individually, drawing out any specific interests they had relative to the project.** I used the information from these one-on-one sessions to assign responsibility to coincide with their interest, allowing me to bring about the best results through a team effort.

RESULT: The feedback from the team was positive. **Everyone felt that he or she made a positive contribution in his or her own distinct way.** It was worth the extra effort I made to listen to each individual and motivate each of them to use their strengths to develop the curriculum.

QUALITY
▶ Communication
▶ Leadership
▶ Ingenuity

DO...

✓ Demonstrate the ability to communicate with a team, and the ability to discuss everyone's strengths to get the most out of their efforts.

✓ Show the committee that you can motivate and persuade people.

DON'T...

✗ Don't talk about being aggressive.

✗ Don't be authoritative, but collaborative.

Give me an example of a time when you took initiative.

As physician assistants we often work autonomously and need to have the ability to take initiative when treating patients. It's okay to contact your supervising physician, but she will not expect you to come to her with every routine problem. You may also be in situations where you must make an instantaneous decision and taking initiative may be the difference between a favorable or a poor patient outcome. Showing your ability to take initiative also instills confidence in your team members.

EXAMPLE ANSWER

SITUATION: This is an example from life outside of my job, but it involves a project that I am very proud of. One day during a meeting after church services, some of the members expressed concern about a homeless woman who frequented the lot next to the church. Winter was approaching and we were concerned that she did not have a warm coat. Some of us had clothes and blankets that we were happy to donate, but we decided this problem was larger than one person.

ACTION: **I suggested that we have a coat drive to see if we could supply coats to as many of the homeless population in our city**

as possible. I volunteered to research the extent of the problem and initiated the coat drive. Some of the church members signed up to help.

RESULT: By the end of the month, we had collected so many coats and blankets that we were able to present them to the homeless woman, as well as various city shelters. Because of our efforts, the mayor of the city presented us with a letter of commendation.

QUALITY

▶ Initiative
▶ Compassion
▶ Empathy
▶ Leadership

DO...

✓ Show that *you* were the one who took the initiative.
✓ Discuss that you also solved the problem using teamwork; under your direction of course.
✓ Notice this example has nothing to do with medicine.

DON'T...

✗ Don't make up a story
✗ Don't give the impression that it was only you who participated.

If you and a colleague or classmate had a personality clash, what would you do to make the relationship better?

The interviewer is probably trying to gauge your professionalism and perseverance, as well as your cooperation skills. The admissions committee is always considering how well you "gel" with your classmates. This is your time to demonstrate to the committee that you have a cooperative style.

EXAMPLE ANSWER

SITUATION: A senior member of our EMT squad tended to criticize my performance in front of staff members during our weekly meetings. He had been a paramedic for over twenty years and he was extremely smart, but his behavior hurt and angered me.

ACTION: Since one of my coworkers, who was a senior EMT, got along well with this senior paramedic, **I took him aside and asked him for an objective appraisal of the situation.** I was surprised when he told me that I had to learn to take criticism better, and although this senior paramedic's manner was harsh, some of his criticisms were justified.

RESULT: **I started working harder in the field to improve my performance.** Soon the senior paramedic was telling me that my performance was improving, and he criticized me less. He also stopped criticizing me in public. He even pulled me aside one day and told me that he was impressed with the improvement I was making. Now, when I receive criticism I take careful notes and use that criticism as a learning tool. I had to persevere and develop a thicker skin, and **I now see criticism as an incentive to improve.**

QUALITY
▶ Not afraid to ask for help
▶ Maturity
▶ Perseverance
▶ Humility
▶ Professionalism
▶ Teachable

DO...

✓ Show that you can take a cooperative approach to problem-solving.

✓ Demonstrate that you are willing and able to seek objective input and bring about objective results—hallmarks of professionalism.

✓ Prove you can use criticism to improve your performance, and that you are able to persevere through negative feedback to find a way to get the job done effectively.

DON'T...

✗ Don't close your mind to criticism when it is delivered in a somewhat harsh way. Instead, look at all situations or criticisms objectively. Ask yourself, "What is my part in this situation?"

✗ Don't hold a resentment toward a supervisor who may give you constructive criticism. Always be positive and draw out a positive result from a negative situation.

Hopefully after seeing some behavioral questions and answers, you will be able to identify a behavioral question, and know how to use the STAR technique to answer them. It is important that you practice answering behavioral questions before your interview.

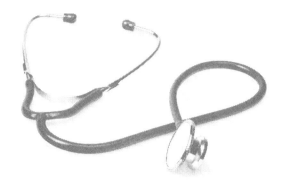

CHAPTER 4

Situational Questions

Your responses to situational questions are extremely important. Situational questions are meant to evaluate many different Qualities. For instance, they are used to...

- ► Elicit specific examples of an applicant's ability to perform under stress.
- ► Evaluate your ability to work collaboratively.
- ► Understand how you will communicate with physicians and other members of the healthcare team.
- ► Assess your problem-solving skills.
- ► Assess your judgment.

As the interviewer finds out more about you and the way you behave in various situations, she will be able to generate a profile of your skillsets, attitudes, and ability to handle a variety of demanding situations.

Target Your Audience

It is always a clever idea to try and tell a story or vignette when answering situational questions. Telling a story will give you more credibility and help you capture the attention of your audience. A key component of telling a story is to keep your audience in mind. You will be interviewing with physician assistants, physician assistant students, faculty members of the PA program, and physicians.

What would you do if you placed an order for a medication in a patient's chart, but the nurse refused to give it?

The interviewer is evaluating your response for a few different qualities:

1. How well can you problem solve?
2. Will you develop an attitude of superiority with the nurse, or will you treat him or her as the colleague he or she really is?
3. Do you place the welfare of your patient above everything else?

EXAMPLE ANSWER

First off, having worked on a medical floor in the hospital, I understand how knowledgeable, professional, and important nurses are to the patients on their floor. **I would not treat this nurse as an adversary, but as a colleague.** Perhaps she knows something that I don't know. I would initially give her the benefit of the doubt, and I certainly wouldn't go over her head without knowing all the facts.

I would approach the nurse and explain that Mr. Jones' potassium is low, and I want to give him enough to bring his potassium up to a safer level. I would then say, **"Am I missing something?"** If the nurse says, "Yes you are. Dr. Smith, the kidney specialist, came up to the floor while you were in another patient's room, and told me not to give potassium to Mr. Jones because he is going for testing this afternoon." In which case I would then say, "Thank you very much (for saving my butt)!"

However, if the nurse couldn't provide me with a plausible reason why she won't give the potassium, **I would have to consider the first rule of medicine, do no harm! I would explain to the nurse**

that I'm concerned that Mr. Jones could possibly have a heart arrhythmia if he doesn't get the potassium. I would advise her, respectfully, that I will ask one of the other nurses to give the potassium. If the other nurse refuses, too, I would call my supervising physician, explain the situation, and allow him to make the final decision.

NOTE: *Based on my personal experience,* please keep in mind that nurses can "make you or break you," depending on how you treat them. Nurses are valuable members of the healthcare team and should be treated as such. Additionally, when you work on a medical floor in a hospital, you become like family. The relationships are collegial and not adversarial. You are all on the same team and these conversations should not be confrontational.

Also, keep in mind that the interviewer may have a hidden motive for asking this question. She may want to see if you are going to use the hierarchical approach: "I'm the PA and you're the nurse. You must follow my orders." Taking that approach would be a huge mistake!

QUALITIES
- ▶ Non-judgmental
- ▶ Collaboration
- ▶ Respect
- ▶ Patient-centered
- ▶ Judgment

DO...
- ✓ Show you are able to consider that your decision may be wrong and keep an open mind.
- ✓ Demonstrate that you believe the nursing staff, and all other ancillary staff, are your colleagues rather than adversaries.
- ✓ Remember that, ultimately, you must consider patient care above all else, and include details that prove that.
- ✓ Show that you know when a situation calls for collaboration with your supervising physician.

DON'T...

✗ Don't imply that the nursing staff are inferior to you.

✗ Don't indicate you make decisions without knowing all the facts.

✗ Don't be afraid to ask for help (from your supervising physician) if appropriate.

You are treating a nine-year-old boy in the emergency room who presented with a fever of 103.5°F, a stiff neck, and vomiting. You are concerned that he may have meningitis and you decide to admit him for a spinal tap in the morning. You present him to one of the ER attendings, who says, "You know we have a bed shortage in the hospital. Send him home and advise his parents to bring him back if he gets any worse."

In this situation, the interviewer is looking to see if you are going to follow the attending's recommendation, just because he is a physician and you're "just" a PA.

EXAMPLE ANSWER

If I felt this patient had meningitis, I would not be comfortable sending him home. He could take a turn for the worse on the drive home, or once he gets home, and he could possibly die before he makes it back to the hospital. I would also have a tough time telling this child's parents that we cannot admit him because of a "bed shortage." That would be totally unacceptable to me, and I'm sure to the patient's parents.

I would try presenting my findings to another attending in the ER to see if she would be willing to admit this child. If she concurred with her colleague, I would have two choices: First, I could call Risk Management (the medical-legal arm of the hospital) and stress the fact that I firmly believe this child is extremely

ill, and that I am concerned he could be contagious and he could possibly die if we send him home. I would also be very clear that a "bed shortage" is no reason to send this patient home. I would ask Risk Management to speak with the attending. Second, I can advise the patient's parents that the attending physician prefers to send their son home and bring him back if he gets worse. However, I would also advise them that I am not in favor of that idea, and I would ask them if they would like me to check another hospital across town to see if they have a bed for him. I would clear this with the attending physician and arrange for EMS transportation.

NOTE: This type of scenario is also presented very often in the PA school interview. Are you going to make a poor decision simply because a physician told you to do so? The committee members are evaluating your maturity and your knowledge of the PA-physician relationship. They will also look to see if you remember that your patient's welfare comes first; "first do no harm."

QUALITIES
▶ Judgment
▶ Problem-solving
▶ Thinking on your feet
▶ Putting the patient's welfare above all else
▶ Maturity

DO...
✓ Trust your clinical judgment.
✓ Advocate for your patient.
✓ Show you are willing to seek out another opinion.
✓ Think outside the box.

DON'T...
✗ Don't compromise your patient's care, or your values, just because you think you cannot challenge "the doctor."
✗ Don't do anything that goes against your judgment and values.

You are on your Ob-Gyn rotation in school, and your supervising physician often leaves you alone to treat patients and sometimes asks you to perform tasks that are outside the scope of practice for a PA student. You really like the rotation and the supervising physician, but you are concerned that you may be crossing the boundaries between student and a licensed practitioner. How would you handle this situation?

As PAs, we typically join a practice and discuss the scope of our practice with the supervising physician. If we feel uncomfortable performing any procedures or tasks, we can meet with our supervising physician and express our concerns. We don't have to worry about flunking a clinical rotation.

As a PA student, we may feel more pressure to keep silent and perform the tasks even though we don't feel comfortable. It can be a difficult and delicate situation to confront your supervising physician or preceptor for fear of getting a poor evaluation on your rotation.

Confronting your supervising physician requires maturity and being true to your values. You would not want to harm a patient if you don't know what you are doing. So, making your feelings known in a mature manner, is a must.

EXAMPLE ANSWER

If I were in this position as a PA student, **I would express my concerns to the supervising physician or my preceptor.** I would first express gratitude for the confidence he has in me. I would go on to explain exactly what I have been doing that is out of the scope of my role as a PA student. **I would express that I feel liable for some of the decisions I am making, and that, as a PA student, I don't feel comfortable accepting that liability.** I would offer to share my program's description of responsibilities and duties that were dictated to us before staring our clinical rotations, and tell him that I am perfectly willing to participate in any of these activities. **I would also tell him that I would not want to jeopardize my standing with the program.**

QUALITIES

▶ Maturity
▶ Integrity
▶ Gratitude
▶ Adhering to your program's rules

DO...

✓ Demonstrate that you remember the first rule of medicine: Do no harm.
✓ Show that you have the maturity to discuss your concerns with your supervising physician or preceptor.
✓ Prove that you are willing to discuss the situation with program faculty if you don't know how to handle the situation.

DON'T...

✗ Don't remain silent and jeopardize patient care or your standing in the program.
✗ Don't be afraid to approach your supervising physician or preceptor with your concerns. You will likely have many similar situations in your career as a PA.
✗ Don't be afraid to ask for help from your program faculty members.

After working a double shift, you realize you gave one of your patients the wrong medication. The patient seems to be doing fine, but you are concerned about your mistake and a possible negative outcome for your patient. What would you do?

This scenario is not as uncommon as you may think. We all make mistakes at one point or another. It's the way you handle your mistakes that makes the difference in the type of provider you will be in the future.

EXAMPLE ANSWER

My first concern would be for my patient's welfare. I would double-check the medication to see if there is a potential for it to harm my patient. I would then speak to the patient directly, informing her that I made a medication error and apologize for the mistake. I would take the patient's vital signs and make sure she is stable. If she appeared to be clinically well, I would advise the patient that it appears the medication did not affect her clinically in any way. **I would address any questions or concerns that she may have relative to the medication error.** I would then document in the patient's chart that I made a medication error, notified the patient, checked her vital signs and clinical status, and addressed any questions or concerns. **I would then notify my supervising physician about the error I made.**

QUALITIES

- ▶ Putting the patient's welfare first
- ▶ Taking responsibility for the mistake
- ▶ Communication with the patient and supervising physician

DO...

✓ Prove that you will place the patient's welfare above all else.
✓ Research possible consequences of giving that medication to the patient.
✓ Show that you are willing to admit to patients when you make a mistake.

DON'T...

✗ Don't ignore the mistake and hope the outcome does no harm.
✗ Don't lie to your patient.
✗ Don't forget this principle; "If you didn't document it, it never happened."
✗ Don't forget to notify your supervising physician.

You have a patient on Medicare and she cannot afford the brand-name medication you prescribed. Medicare will not cover the medication until she has failed two generic medications first. The patient approaches you asking you to contact the insurance company and advise them she already failed the two generics (even though she hasn't), so she can get the brand-name medication. What would you do?

Insurance companies frequently deny brand-name medications due to the expense of the drug. Typically, the insurance company will ask for a prior authorization (PA) before they will prescribe the brand-name. Usually this is as simple as completing a form or even just checking off a box on the form stating the patient meets the requirements for the brand-name medication. By signing this Federal document, the provider assumes responsibility of meeting Medicare's criteria.

EXAMPLE ANSWER

This is a situation that could be very uncomfortable, especially if the patient is very persistent. **I would not sign the prior authorization paperwork and I would not prescribe the brand-name medication.** I would explain to the patient that she may do very well on the generic medication, which would save both her and the government a lot of money. I would also explain to her that if I sign the prior authorization paperwork, **I would be committing Medicare fraud.** I could face severe punishment, and I will not risk my medical license.

QUALITIES

▶ Integrity
▶ Reasoning
▶ Maturity
▶ Ethics
▶ Judgment

DO...

✓ Demonstrate understanding of ethics.
✓ Show willingness to offer an alternative option.
✓ Explain to the patient the negative consequences of committing Medicare fraud; including the fact that it could result in you losing your license.
✓ *Always* do the right thing.

DON'T...

✗ Don't insinuate that you would commit fraud.
✗ Don't imply that you would jeopardize your medical license, even if a patient is persistent.

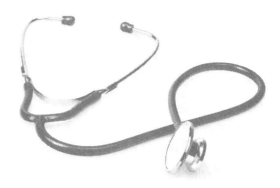

CHAPTER 5

Ethical Questions

What Are Ethical Issues?

Ethical issues are problems or dilemmas involving moral compromise. They can arise anywhere. They can be thought of on a societal scale, like, "Should federal funding be withheld from sanctuary cities?" or on an individual level, like, "Does a priest have the right to refuse marrying a same-sex couple?"

The Eight Most Common Ethical Scenarios

During your PA school interview(s,) you are very likely to be asked one or more ethical questions as they relate to health care. In my experience working with thousands of PA school applicants, the following topics are a typical source of medical ethical questions:

- Abortion
- Managed care
- Patient confidentiality
- Refusal and withdrawal of treatment

- Genetic testing
- Cheating on a test
- Medical malpractice

If you had to choose to give a liver transplant either to a successful, and otherwise-healthy, seventy-two-year-old female member of the community, or a twenty-year-old male who is an active alcoholic and drug addict, who would you choose to receive the liver and why?

The key to answering this question is to not be judgmental. You want to make your decision strictly on the medical facts. Discuss both sides of the argument and show your interviewer that your decision is not being made on any type of bias, like age or social status.

EXAMPLE ANSWER

I would choose to give this "gift" to the seventy-two-year-old female.

Even though, at first glance, the twenty-one-year-old male would seem to have many more years of life to live, I would need to, non-judgmentally, consider the **facts** as you laid out in this question.

The twenty-year-old male is an **active** alcoholic and drug addict, which means he continues to drink and use drugs while waiting for a liver transplant. **I would not simply assume that he would get clean and sober after the surgery. If he is on a transplant list and still using, he is clearly not ready to quit his destructive behavior.**

Additionally, after a transplant surgery, the recipient would need to be on anti-rejection medications for life and would need to be compliant with multiple follow-up visits with the transplant team. **I believe if he is still actively using drugs and alcohol, his body would be more likely to reject the liver in a matter of weeks or months.**

On the other hand, there is no mention of any lifestyle changes in the seventy-two-year-old female that would compromise her acceptance of the liver. Even if she gets ten years of life after the liver transplant, that would be much longer than weeks or months, as would likely be the case with the twenty-year-old active addict.

I would imagine the person who donated this precious gift would want the donor to be someone who will cherish it and live a healthy life to enjoy its benefits for as long as possible.

QUALITIES
- ▶ Decisive
- ▶ Insight
- ▶ Non-judgmental
- ▶ Reasoning
- ▶ Considers issue from both sides

DO...
- ✓ Show you can consider the pros and cons of each patient.
- ✓ Think about the long-term consequences of your decision, and make sure your answer reflects that.
- ✓ Explain that you understand a donated organ is a precious item that requires careful considerations.

DON'T...
- ✘ Don't be judgmental when explaining your decision.
- ✘ Don't show naivety and assume the hypothetical younger patient will magically get clean and sober if he is the recipient of the liver. Explain that if he had been sober for a year before the transplant, that might change your decision
- ✘ Don't tell your interviewer that you would never have to make that type of decision

Would you assist a physician in performing an abortion?

The topic of abortion has clearly become a political battlefield in this country. The last thing you want to do is discuss politics at your PA school interview. If you agree to assist on an abortion, you will be labeled as "pro-choice." If you do not agree to assist on the abortion, you will be labeled as "pro-life." Depending on the politics of the interviewer, the wrong answer can be risky. So how do you answer this question without giving away your politics? Let's look.

EXAMPLE ANSWER

If I were pro-choice, I would have no problem assisting a physician in an abortion. If I were pro-life, I would not take a job where I might be in that situation.

QUALITIES

▶ Remains apolitical
▶ Avoids controversy

DO...

✓ Consider what the "question behind the question" may be and choose the appropriate response.
✓ Recognize the question as a political one.
✓ Avoid political discussions at all costs

DON'T...

✗ Don't choose an answer that you think the committee wants to hear.
✗ Don't rush your answer. Think about the potential consequences of your answer.
✗ Don't give away your political persuasion.

You are a cardiac surgery PA. A forty-year-old male was recently brought into the ER with crushing chest pain. The patient had a cardiac catheterization, and his cardiologist decided he needs an urgent cardiac bypass surgery. Your job is to go to the ER, perform a quick history and physical examination, then have the patient sign a consent form accepting the risks and benefits of the surgery.

You go down to the emergency room and meet this very pleasant male, and note that he is of sound mind and in good spirits. You complete a quick history and physical, and then begin to go over the consent form. You start advising the patient of some potential risks of cardiac surgery; death, stroke, bleeding which may require a blood transfusion, etc. The patient tells you that he is a Jehovah Witness, and it is against his religion to receive a blood transfusion. You explain to the patient that bleeding is very common, and he may need a transfusion to save his life. The patient again refuses, so you take him to the OR and advise the surgeon that the patient refuses a blood transfusion, if necessary.

The patient does very well in the operating room and you bring him to the intensive care unit. As soon as you transfer him from the stretcher to his bed, he starts to crash. His blood pressure drops, his heart rate speeds up, and his EKG tracing shows that he is going into a potentially fatal arrhythmia. You glance at his chest tube container and notice he is bleeding profusely. He needs a blood transfusion to save his life. What would you do?

In my personal role as a cardiac surgery PA, I faced this very dilemma multiple times. It is not an unusual situation. The decisions we make can be very difficult at times because we are trained to always do our best to save lives. However, we must also be acutely aware of medical-legal issues. If a patient has a Do Not Resuscitate (DNR) order, do we have the right to resuscitate that patient because we don't want him to die? No, we don't. Although you may feel helpless watching someone die, you have no right to overrule a patient's expressed wishes.

EXAMPLE ANSWER

Admittedly, this would be a very difficult situation.

The first thing I would do would be to have one of the nurses call the surgeon and notify her that the patient is crashing. **I would do everything in my power to support the patient, including IV fluids, medications to maintain his blood pressure, anti-arrhythmia medications, and check for the source of bleeding.**

I would not give blood products! The patient was of sound mind when he signed the consent form, and I could not ethically go against his wishes.

QUALITIES
▶ Empathy
▶ Resourceful
▶ Ethical

DO...
✓ Show you are willing to respect the patient's wishes, even though it may not be the best course of action from a strict medical perspective.
✓ Show you understand your medical-legal obligations.
✓ Indicate you would try to keep the patient alive by using all available resources, aside from those that violate the wishes of the patient.

DON'T...

✘ Don't imply you will make your decision based on *your own* beliefs.

✘ Don't be overly emotional in your response.

✘ Don't forget to contact the surgeon!

Have you ever been in a situation at work, or in school, where you felt it was necessary to address an ethical issue? Describe the situation.

The way you handle ethical issues tells a lot about your character, integrity, and maturity. In medicine, ethical issues come up all the time. You must be able to do the "right thing," and not take the easy way out because you don't like confrontation.

EXAMPLE ANSWER

I was in college taking an examination in biochemistry. I noticed a student who was sitting in the bottom row using small notes written in blue ink on the palms of both hands. He kept referring to the notes before answering questions.

I would approach the student after class, and say, "**I feel** like you were cheating on the exam. I see you have notes on your hand, and I saw you referring to them. Were you cheating?

If the student acknowledged that he was cheating, I would first ask him why. If he told me he was having some personal problems, or he found the information to be very difficult, **I would offer to help him study.**

I would then explain to the student that, by cheating, he is harming his classmates who took the time to study; grades may be based on a curve. I would also explain that if he doesn't know the material, he could potentially harm a patient in the future.

Finally, although it would be difficult, and may jeopardize my classmate's future in the class, I would be forced to do the right thing. I would advise the student that I will give him three choices: tell the professor he was cheating, allow me to go to the professor with him, or that I will tell the professor myself if he doesn't follow through with the first two choices.

QUALITIES

- ▶ Maturity
- ▶ Non-accusatory (I 'feel" like you may have been cheating; feelings aren't facts)
- ▶ Compassion
- ▶ Ethical
- ▶ Leadership
- ▶ Ability to do the *right thing*

DO...

- ✓ Stand up for your beliefs.
- ✓ Show that you are assertive, but not aggressive.
- ✓ Show that you are compassionate
- ✓ Always think about others; your classmates and especially future patients.

DON'T...

- ✗ Don't choose a story in which you were aggressive, rather than assertive.
- ✗ Don't use language that may come across as vindictive.
- ✗ Don't accuse, gather information first.

What would you do if you caught your colleague stealing controlled medications?

In a real scenario, this is a difficult ethical dilemma. Your colleague may be a good friend, and reporting her to your supervising physician may jeopardize her career. On the other hand, you know that you cannot ignore the situation.

EXAMPLE ANSWER

Stealing drugs is a serious offense and should not be taken lightly. **The first thing I'd do is convince my colleague to put the drugs back immediately.** I would sit her down in private and ask her why she is stealing the medication. I would tell her that since I know she is stealing drugs, she is putting my license, our supervising physician's license, and her entire career in jeopardy.

If she told me she was stealing the drugs to give to a friend or a relative who may not have insurance, **I would advise her that there are alternative ways to get medication legally.** I would point out to her that many pharmaceutical companies may offer her the medication for free. I would then advise her of the consequences if her friend or relative had an allergic reaction or overdosed and died.

I would consider other reasons why she may feel the need to steal controlled drugs. Was she struggling with addiction? Was she selling the drugs for money? If she admitted to having a problem with addiction, I would offer to help her any way I could. If she was stealing the drugs for money, I would probably have a lot less tolerance.

Finally, I would feel compelled to discuss this situation with my supervising physician. Again, if I didn't, I could jeopardize my job or my medical license. I might speak with the physician and propose a hypothetical question about this sort of dilemma, and what the right thing to do would be. I would accept whatever advice she gave.

QUALITIES

▶ Ethical
▶ Empathy
▶ Judgment
▶ Assertive
▶ Doing the right thing

DO...

✓ Make sure your answer reflects that you understand how serious this situation is.
✓ Show that you would be nonjudgmental and listen to what your colleague has to say.
✓ Explain that you would need to discuss the situation with your supervising physician.
✓ Be assertive, not aggressive

DON'T...

✗ Don't indicate that you would look the other way in this situation.
✗ Don't jeopardize your medical license because she is your colleague.
✗ Don't let her leave the floor with the drugs

You typically call all your patients back with lab results. One day you call Mr. Jones to advise him about a finding on one of his labs. Mrs. Jones answers the phone and tells you that Mr. Jones is not home. She then says, "It's okay, you can give me the results and I'll pass them on to him." What would you do in this situation?

It is quite common to call patients daily and discuss their recent lab work or test results. Often the patient is not home, and the spouse answers the phone and says, "You can give me the results and I'll let him know." The spouse may also ask, "Is there anything wrong?" Knowing how to handle these situations is extremely important; but the answer is quite straightforward.

EXAMPLE ANSWER

This scenario sounds to me like a HIPPA concern. It seems to be a cut-and-dried issue. I would explain to Mrs. Jones that I cannot give her the results because it would be a HIPPA violation. If the results are normal, **I would reassure her that everything is okay, and I'm just making a routine call to give Mr. Jones his test results.** I would also ask Mrs. Jones to have her husband call me back when he gets home.

QUALITIES

- ▶ Knowledge of HIPPA regulations
- ▶ Empathy
- ▶ Integrity

DO...

- ✓ Demonstrate understanding of HIPPA.
- ✓ Be empathetic with the spouse but stick to your values.

DON'T...

- ✗ Don't consider violating HIPPA, even if you know the spouse very well.

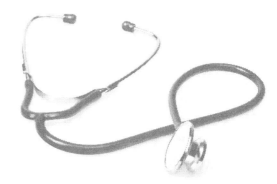

CHAPTER 6

Illegal Questions

Like a professor preparing good test questions, selecting appropriate interview questions is a skill. It is important to keep in mind that although professors write test questions for a living, PA school admissions committee members are not always professional interviewers. ADCOM members are often graduates of the program who have no formal experience conducting interviews. As a result, these committee members may ask "illegal" interview questions.

A common misconception is that people believe it is illegal for these questions to be asked. That is not the case. It is not against the law to ask these questions, but it *is* illegal for an interviewer to take the response into account during hiring (under the Equal Employment Opportunity Commission), and could open them up to a lawsuit if an applicant files a complaint. Therefore, it's in the best interest of the interviewer to not ask, or the interviewee not to answer.

If you are asked one of these interview questions, don't become defensive. Ask yourself, "Do I want to be right, or do I want to be effective?

To be effective, versus being right, I recommend that you assume the interviewer asked the question out of ignorance, and not to trip you up. The good news is that you don't have to answer these questions directly. There is always a hidden question behind the question.

As you will see, there is a way to deflect the question and address the *real* question behind it.

Here is a list of questions where the response would be illegal to take into consideration by the admissions or hiring committee:

▸ Questions about marital or family status

▸ Questions about age

▸ Questions about disabilities

▸ Questions about national origin/citizenship

▸ Questions about military service

▸ Questions about political affiliations

▸ Questions about race/color/religion

Now, let's look at some actual questions and answers...

Do you have any children?

The interviewer may ask this question as a way of "fortune telling." The underlying question is probably, "Will you be missing classes and clinical rotation days because your children may be sick, and you don't have day care?"

The best way to answer this question is:

There is nothing in my family situation that will interfere with my ability to attend class or clinical rotations.

Comparable questions to consider:

▸ Are you married?

▸ Are you planning to have children?

▸ Are you pregnant?

▸ Do you have day care available?

How old are you?

This question is probably more about maturity than chronological age. The best way to answer this question is:

I've accomplished all the academic prerequisites and the required number of clinical hours to qualify for this program. I know what it takes to become a good physician assistant, and I am ready to embrace the challenges of PA school.

Comparable questions to consider:

- ▸ When were you born?
- ▸ What is your date of birth?

How much do you weigh?

This is a rude interview question, to say the least. The interviewer may be thinking you may not be able to handle the job as a PA if you are overweight or obese. Or, if you're very thin, the interviewer may think you have anorexia and may be hospitalized at some point during the program.

The interviewer may also have a bias toward overweight or obese applicants.

The best way to answer this question is:

Weight has never been an issue for me. I've never had a problem performing any of my job duties.

Comparable questions to consider:

- ▸ "How tall are you?"
- ▸ "Do you exercise?"

I see you're not moving your arm very well; did you hurt yourself?

This is a *fishing* question to see if you have a disability that might interfere with your duties as a PA.

The best way to answer this question is:

I'm fine, thank you.

No need to elaborate!

Comparable questions to consider:

▶ What medications do you take?

▶ Do you have any mental health issues?

▶ Do you have heart disease?

▶ Have you ever been treated for alcoholism or drug addiction?

▶ Do you have an eating disorder?

▶ Will you need us to make accommodations for you to complete the program?

You have an interesting accent. What country are you from?

Inquiries about an applicant's citizenship or country of birth could imply discrimination based on national origin.

The best way to answer this question is:

I'm an American citizen.

Comparable questions to consider:

▶ Where were you born?

▶ Are you a citizen of this country?

▶ Your last name sounds Italian, is it?

Have you ever been arrested?

Upon completion of PA school, you will undergo a background check to see if you qualify for a medical license. If you have any felonies or drug convictions, you will be disqualified. You may want to consider this before applying. However, if you have been arrested for any minor offenses but not convicted, you don't have to divulge that information. If you have a current arrest, the admissions committee can ask you about that and take it into consideration when deciding on your candidacy.

The best way to answer this question is (if appropriate):

No. I've never been convicted of a criminal offense.

Comparable questions to consider:

▸ Have you ever committed a crime?

Have you ever served in the military, or are you currently on active duty or in the reserves?

Even though the first PA school class was made up of former U.S. Navy corpsman, don't assume that all committee members are pro-military.

If your military training is relevant and supportive of your application to PA school, you may want to elaborate on the specifics of your training and your job duties. However, be cautious about your answers and about divulging too much information.

There is one exception to this rule: If the program has a quota for veterans, be sure to let them know you've served the country.

The best way to answer this question is:

Yes, I received an honorable discharge from the Navy in 2001. Or, No, I did not serve.

Are you a Republican or a Democrat?

This is a *loaded* question. Never discuss politics at an interview unless you want to sabotage your chances of being accepted. People usually have strong feelings about their political persuasion and you wouldn't want to make your interviewer angry.

The best way to answer this question is:

It is my policy never to discuss politics with my friends, and certainly not at a PA school interview.

Comparable questions to consider:

▸ Who did you vote for in the last election?

▸ Are you in a union?

▸ What do you think about the president?

What religion are you?

Interviewers may ask you about your religious background to see if you will have any conflict working Saturdays or Sundays.

The best way to answer this question is:

My religious views are very personal.

Comparable questions to consider:

▸ Are you Caucasian/African American/Hispanic?

▸ Do you attend church/temple/a Mosque?

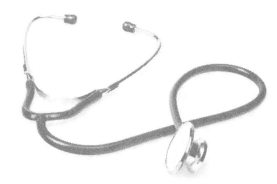

CHAPTER 7

The MMI Interview

In previous chapters, we've covered almost every possible question that you might be asked at your PA school interview. However, some of you may be notified that your upcoming interview is going to be in a much different format than a traditional interview. You may be taking part in a Multiple Mini Interview, or MMI. Chances are you've never even heard of the MMI-style interview, let alone participated in one.

A small percentage of applicants I've spoken with, after having an MMI interview, rate the MMI as being more difficult than traditional interviews. Most of these applicants also admit they did not prepare for the MMI format, and naturally didn't do very well.

In this chapter, I'm going to cover:

- ▸ What is the MMI?
- ▸ How to approach the MMI.
- ▸ How to answer MMI questions.
- ▸ Review of key points.

There are an infinite number of prompts that you may be asked/ given at an MMI interview. Therefore, this chapter will not contain multiple questions with sample answers. Rather, I am going to cover the four points above, and use one single prompt as an example of how to approach and answer MMI questions.

What Is the MMI?

The MMI format, is the newest type of interview being utilized by PA programs. This interview format is considered by some PA programs to be a better indicator of academic and clinical performance. The MMI better assesses the candidate's nonacademic qualities and the ability to think on her feet.

History of the MMI

In 2004, the Michael DeGroote School of Medicine at McMaster University (Canada) began developing the MMI format to address two widely recognized problems:

1. Traditional interview formats do not accurately predict performance in medical school.
2. The most common patient complaints relate to non-cognitive skills, such as interpersonal skills, professionalism, and ethical/moral judgment.

McMaster has reported that the use of the MMI has increased the reliability of the interview in assessing a candidate's suitability for the practice of medicine.

Format of the MMI

During an MMI, the interviewee moves from station to station during a designated time- period throughout the day. The stations are simply interview rooms that may be lined up in a hallway, or in a circular fashion. Once the applicant completes station one, she moves on to station two. The applicant keeps progressing until she's completed all the designated stations. The number of stations will vary from program to program.

Some interviews are occasionally split interviews, with half of the interview in the MMI format, and the other half in a traditional format. Typically, you can expect a full MMI interview to last approximately two hours, with breaks.

There are typically six-to-eight stations during an MMI interview. The interviewee is given anywhere from six to ten minutes to complete a station.

Upon arrival at a station, you will find a note card or piece of paper on the door, with a written prompt on it. The prompt may consist of:

- A scenario that you must discuss when you enter the room.
- A task you must complete inside of the room.
- A role-playing scenario.
- A scenario that involves another student or administrator.

You will have two minutes outside of the room to read the prompt and begin to formulate your response. You may be able to take notes, but it is not guaranteed. This is something you will want to find out *before* your interview date.

After the two-minute time frame is up, a bell will sound, notifying you that it is time to enter the interview room to discuss the prompt with the interviewer.

Once inside the room, you will have from four to eight minutes (depending on the length of the station) to complete your response.

Let's review the sequence of events during an MMI station:

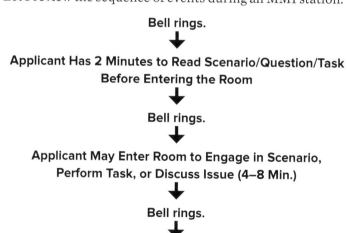

Bell rings.

↓

Applicant Has 2 Minutes to Read Scenario/Question/Task Before Entering the Room

↓

Bell rings.

↓

Applicant May Enter Room to Engage in Scenario, Perform Task, or Discuss Issue (4–8 Min.)

↓

Bell rings.

↓

End of Time Period. Applicant Proceeds To Next Station*

*The process continues until the applicant completes all stations.

TIP: Be sure to wear a watch when you come for your interview. Most likely, there will not be a clock in the hallway or inside the room. The last thing you want to have happen is having the bell go off inside the room when you are trying to wrap up an answer. When the bell rings, you stop!

Goal of the MMI

The goal of the MMI is to assess your nonacademic qualities, and your ability to think and react quickly.

Why MMI Over Traditional Interview?

To assess nonacademic qualities. Your many Qualities may be assessed at each of the stations in the MMI. See the chart on the opposite page for a list of Qualities most assessed by admissions committees.

There Are No Right or Wrong Answers

Applicants are all graded on a spectrum, which allows for better comparison of candidates.

MMIs Minimize Examiner Bias

- ▸ Multiple independent assessors and stations
- ▸ Flexibility in scenarios
- ▸ Allows for recovery in a disastrous station

Why Is the MMI Important?

Most applicants selected for a PA school interview have high GPAs, excellent test scores, and a great deal of medical experience. The MMI is a way to distinguish yourself from the other highly qualified applicants. Once you reach your interview, it can be the single most important aspect of your application.

Personal Characteristics Assessed During the Admissions Interview

Characteristics	Percentage
Motivation for a medical career	98%
Compassion and empathy	96%
Personal maturity	92%
Oral communication	91%
Service orientation	89%
Professionalism	88%
Altruism (selflessness)	83%
Integrity	82%
Leadership	80%
Intellectual curiosity	76%
Teamwork	74%
Cultural competence	72%
Reliability and dependability	70%
Self-discipline	70%
Critical thinking	69%
Adaptability	67%
Verbal reasoning	66%
Work habits	66%
Persistence	65%
Resilience	65%
Logical reasoning	56%

Source: Adapted from the Association of American Medical Colleges (AAMC), www.aamc.org.

How to Approach the MMI

At each station, the interviewee is asked to respond to one of the following prompts. You will need to know *what* to say, and *how* to say it. Here are a few common prompts that you may receive:

- ► Ethical dilemma
- ► Knowledge of PA profession/healthcare
- ► Role-playing scenarios
- ► Task station

Example of an Ethical Dilemma

An attending physician is in the habit of introducing PAs rotating with him as "Doctors." Discuss the ethical issues raised by this practice.

Example of Knowledge of the PA Profession

Talk about Full Practice Authority and Responsibility (FPAR) as it relates to the PA profession. Are you for FPAR or against it? How do you think it will change the PA profession?

NOTE: *If you do not know what Full Practice Authority and Responsibility (FPAR) means to the PA profession, Google "AAPA Task Force and FPAR" for a summary.*

Example of Role-Playing Scenario

You work in a family practice clinic. The next patient on your schedule is Mr. Jones. You must inform Mr. Jones that his recent CT scan shows that he has cancer in his pancreas with metastases to other parts of his body. How would you break the sad news?

Example of a Task Station

You walk into the station and you find a pair of sterile gloves on the table and instructions for putting them on. In a separate part of the room, isolated from you, is another student who also has a pair of sterile gloves on the table in front of her. Your task is to teach/explain to the other applicant how to put the gloves on in a sterile fashion.

The interviewer(s) will observe and score your performance. All of the interviewees will be presented the same exact questions, scenarios, and tasks for consistency. Keep in mind that in an MMI interview, you can see any number of prompts. Here are some other examples of MMI prompts you may encounter.

- Discuss your past experiences with PAs.
- Why are you a good fit for the PA profession? Please discuss your qualifications and experiences.
- What are your biggest strengths and weaknesses?
- Write a letter to a professor about a bad grade (D+) you received on your final paper of the semester. Note that the professor's comments state that your grammar was an issue and the analysis of the topic was superficial.
- *Anatomy station:* Write out the flow of blood through the systemic circulation starting with the Inferior Vena Cava.
- *Anatomy station:* You will be given an anterior and posterior view of the knee. Label as many structures as you can.
- *Role playing:* You are a phlebotomist in a hospital. Treat this room as if you are with a patient with whom you struggled to get blood. You must retake more blood because you drew the original sample into the wrong colored tube. How would you deal with this situation? Also, describe the difference between sympathy and empathy.
- If one student in your group project cheated, should all the students in the group fail?
- You must choose a punishment, and level of punishment, for a professional infraction. For *type* of punishment, the choices include:
  - Verbal warning
  - Written warning
  - Probation
  - Dismissal

For *level* of punishment your choices are:

- Mild
- Moderate
- Severe
- None

The infractions include:

- Dishonesty
- Informally addressing a superior
- Plagiarism

As you can see from the examples above, there are any number of prompts that you may have to address at your MMI interview. One issue that you may come across is fatigue from the volume of prompts you will be discussing on interview day. I strongly recommend that you practice MMI scenarios a few weeks before your actual interview. You can start with one per day for a week, then increase the number of prompts and answers at your own pace. I recommend that you increase the number of prompts until you can answer six to eight prompts in one sitting.

Do not try to memorize answers or practice scenarios; there is too much variation between the different programs.

Failure to prepare, is preparing to fail. —Benjamin Franklin

Responding to an MMI Prompt

- ▸ What to say
- ▸ How to say it

What to Say in Your Response

- ▸ **The Four Pillars of Medical Ethics**

  1. **Autonomy** refers to the capacity to think, decide, and act on one's own free initiative. The concept of the PA profession is based on this principle.

2. **Beneficence** (charity mercy, kindness) involves promoting what is best for the patient given all viable options and complicating factors.

3. **Non-maleficence** (non-harming) refers to the principle of *first do no harm and* may be encompassed under beneficence.

4. **Justice** is the science and art of prioritizing the distribution of limited resources

▸ **Professional Competency Roles**
   - Professional
   - Communicator
   - Manager
   - Health advocate
   - Scholar
   - Healthcare system/training in the field
   - Almost all prompts can be related to healthcare
   - Show how you could apply a scenario to healthcare

EXAMPLE: How to incorporate the healthcare system into your response.

Healthcare System: The prompt asks you what you would do if you walked out of your front door one day and found a shoebox with $100,000 in it. There is no note, and no identifying information on the box.

At first glance, it's not obvious how you might bring the healthcare system into this discussion. If not done properly, your answer can seem forced and off-point.

It takes a lot of practice and thinking on your feet to incorporate these points strategically, and may not be appropriate for every scenario.

RESPONSE

After providing a full answer to the prompt question, you could add the following:

> While the decision-making process in this example is challenging, I would imagine that healthcare providers are faced with even greater challenges every day. Here I might have to advise a patient that there are many courses of treatment to consider for his illness, each having pros and cons.
>
> I would approach the conversation regarding treatment options using similar strategies that I discussed when making the appropriate decision on what to do with the money.

Connecting a general prompt to healthcare is a wonderful way to highlight your potential as a PA student and as a professional.

It is also a great idea to incorporate some of your past individual experiences when answering the prompt.

Responding well to a hypothetical ethical scenario is great but *demonstrating* that you've had success using these techniques in the real world can make your answer even stronger, and in some cases, more compelling.

Let's build off our example above on deciding what to do with the $100,000 you found on your doorstep. After answering the question, you may want to bring in a personal experience.

EXAMPLE: How to incorporate a personal experience into your prompt.

> After graduating college, I joined a church group. One day a single mom joined the group and it was obvious she was struggling with finances. She had recently been living in a shelter with her three children and was struggling to feed and clothe them. One day I decided to purchase a bunch of groceries for her, and clothes for the kids. I left the packages on her front step and left. I've always liked doing things for people and not getting caught.

By relating the prompts to your own experiences, you prove to the interviewer that you possess the Qualities that are valuable to a competent medical provider. Learning to incorporate the healthcare system and personal experiences into the answers to prompts takes a great deal of practice.

How to Say It: Strategies for Dealing with a Prompt

Now that we have discussed what to say when responding to an MMI prompt, let's explore how to say it. Here are four strategies for dealing with a prompt:

1. Know what the prompt is asking. The worst thing you can do is *not* answer the question. Many applicants I coach do this a lot when I ask them the question, "Why do you want to become a PA?" They tell me "I've always been fascinated by science," "I love helping people," and that they are a "team player." They never answer the specific question, "Why do you want to become a PA?" The answers above could be relevant to becoming a paramedic, nurse, physician, or a medical assistant.

2. Manage your time. It is going to take a considerable amount of practice to answer a prompt in six or eight minutes. Again, make sure you wear a watch to the interview. With an infinite number of possible prompts and the stress surrounding the MMI, it's natural to become nervous about this process. It is also very important to learn how to manage your anxiety. Having a structure in place to answer the prompts will go a long way to calm your nerves.

   When you first start practicing answering MMI prompts, you are probably going to find that you will not be able to fill the time. Then, as you practice a little more, you'll probably find that you have too much to talk about. At this point you are well practiced at viewing prompts from different perspectives. Now is when you need to learn to focus on the most salient points.

3. Formulate a strategy for answering the prompt. It is imperative to have a strategy for breaking down a prompt into its most important parts. It also gives structure for how to develop and deliver your content in a timely manner.

   I find the best strategy for answering a prompt is to:
   - First identify the issues/actors and missing information.
   - Consider the issues from multiple perspectives before stating your answer.
   - End effectively.

   (Later in this chapter, I'll illustrate how to use this strategy by providing examples.)

4. Listen for feedback and follow up prompts from your interviewer. The interviewer may ask you follow up questions. This is a great opportunity to turn a monologue into a dialogue.

In addition, interviewers may have their own questions they want to ask at the end of your response, or throughout your response. This tests your ability to listen and is also an opportunity for you to showcase your ability to adapt to additional information.

Being an effective listener is a Quality that you will need to be an effective clinician. You must listen to your patients, and not just talk to them.

How to Answer MMI Questions

Let's now look at an MMI prompt and how to answer it using what we've learned so far.

Outside the Room (2–3 minutes)

EXAMPLE PROMPT

It has been long debated in the PA profession whether to change the name of the profession from *physician assistant* to *physician associate*. Many PAs feel that the word *assistant* does not accurately reflect the advanced training and abilities that PAs have, and they feel patients may mistake them as medical assistants. If you frequent the PA Forum (physicianassistantforum.com), you will find a variety of comments on this topic. Most favor changing the name to Physician Associate. In a small poll posted on Inside PA Training's website (mypatraining.com), 507 participants voted on this topic. Here are the results:

- ► 360 participants (71.01%) voted to change the name to "physician associate"
- ► 79 participants (15.58%) voted not to change the name
- ► 60 participants (13.41%) voted to change the name, but not to "physician associate"

If you had the tie-breaking vote on choosing to keep the name or change the name, how would you vote and why? Would you change the name to physician associate? Would you change the name to something else? Would you keep the name as it is? Who should be considered before making your decision?

Questions to Think About

1. Do *you* think that physician assistants should vote to change the name of the profession to "physician associate?"
2. Should PAs vote to change the name, or keep it the same?
3. Should PAs vote to choose a different name for the PA profession?
4. What is *your* opinion on changing the name?
5. Who should be consulted/considered when making this decision?

Set a timer for two minutes and prepare your response.

This exercise may seem completely overwhelming at first. Don't worry! This is most likely the first time you've had to answer an MMI prompt and formulating a response to this answer in two minutes is a challenging task. You may be thinking, "How am I going to plan an eight-minute response in two or three minutes?" The answer is to read on, and practice, practice, practice.

With more practice, it will make it much easier to plan what you'd like to say, inside the room, in such a brief time frame.

Inside the Room (6–8 minutes)

SUMMARIZE THE PROMPT

Always start with a summary of the prompt. You want to make sure that you understand the prompt correctly, and that you're on the same page with the interviewer. By asking, "Do I have this right?" at the end of your summary, you'll get the dialogue started with the interviewer.

EXAMPLE

Let's look at a possibility for a summary statement:

I have been asked to discuss my thoughts about considering a name change for the PA profession. The question is about whether PAs should change the name of the profession to "physician associate," keep the name as it is, or vote to change the name to something other than "physician associate." The prompt is also asking my opinion on the topic and who should be consulted or considered about the name change. Do I have this correct?

Summarizing the prompt is also a terrific way to "break the ice." It could be very intimidating if you're in the room for six to eight minutes with an interviewer who is silent and unresponsive.

More importantly, starting with the summary of the prompt and asking, "Do I have this right?" is a wonderful way to know if you may have interpreted the prompt differently than the interviewer.

I now want you to go back to the above prompt and summarize the key points in fifteen seconds. Set a timer and see how well you do.

- ► Should PAs vote to change the name of the PA profession to Physician Associate?
- ► Should PAs keep the name as it is?
- ► Should PAs vote to choose a different name for the PA profession?

- ▸ What is your opinion on changing the name?
- ▸ Who should be consulted/considered concerning the name change?

Notice how succinct the summary is, and how it gets right to the point. I bet that was a lot simpler than you thought it would be. When you ask the interviewer, "Do I have this correct?" you start a dialogue, and you can rest assured you're on the right track.

Once you summarize the prompt, the next step is to employ your strategy for answering the prompt. I recommend a strategy that you've already used when writing a traditional six-paragraph essay. Start with an opening statement, which would be equivalent to your opening paragraph in an essay.

In this case, the introduction should include identifying the actors/issues, and any missing information. Also, you should determine if there are any ethical considerations. It is a good idea to explicitly state this information, so the interviewer understands your thought process. The introductory paragraph should also include a mini-outline for the rest of your answer. It tells the interviewer what you are going to discuss in the remainder of your answer. The last sentence should also contain a transitional "hook," which takes you to the body of your answer.

Next, use a few paragraphs for the body of your answer. Use a topic sentence and a few sentences to support your topic sentence, and then use a transition sentence to take you to the next paragraph. Use three or four paragraphs in the body of your answer. Finally, end the answer with a strong summary/conclusion.

Explicitly identify the key players who are involved in the scenario and any participants who will be affected by any action that the players take.

Provide the Body of Your Answer

The body of your answer is where we identify:

- ▸ Key actors and stakeholders who are involved in the scenario.
- ▸ Missing information or unknown parts of the prompt.
  - Be strategic—don't give a laundry list
  - Ask for clarification.
  - Make assumptions and continue.

Here is the same prompt again. Try to find the actors, missing information, and key issues.

EXAMPLE

It has been long debated in the PA profession whether to change the name of the profession from *physician assistant* to *physician associate*. Many PAs feel that the word *assistant* does not accurately reflect the advanced training and abilities that PAs have, and they feel patients may mistake them as medical assistants. If you frequent the PA Forum (physicianassistantforum.com), you will find a variety of comments on this topic. Most favor changing the name to Physician Associate. In a small poll posted on Inside PA Training's website (mypatraining.com,) 507 participants voted on this topic. Here are the results:

- ▸ 360 participants (71.01%) voted to change the name to "physician associate"
- ▸ 79 participants (15.58%) voted not to change the name
- ▸ 60 participants (13.41%) voted to change the name, but not to "physician associate"

If you had the tie-breaking vote on choosing to keep the name or change the name, how would you vote and why? Would you change the name to physician associate? Would you change the name to something else? Would you keep the name as it is? Who should be considered before making your decision?

The Actors, the Missing Information, and the Issues

▶ Should PA students, as well as practicing PAs, be allowed to vote on a name change? Would a much larger sample of voters yield the same results as the small sample used in the above poll?

▶ What about PA program faculty? Should they have a vote?

▶ How would physicians react to the name change?

What About the Public?

▶ How well would patients accept the name change?

▶ Would patients become confused by a name change?

▶ How long would it take to reeducate patients?

▶ Would a name change improve patient satisfaction?

▶ Is a name change about ego, or clarity of the profession?

What About the Profession Itself?

▶ The Bureau of Labor Statistics (BLS) projects the PA profession to grow 37% from 2016–2026. Would the growth rate increase because of a name change?

▶ The BLS has consistently ranked the PA profession as one of the top career fields. Would changing the name increase the ranking of the profession?

▶ Would PA salaries increase due to a name change?

▶ Would PAs be more respected by other healthcare providers with a name change?

Logistics of a Name Change

How much money would be needed to change the name of the profession? A name change would financially impact every PA program, the American Academy of Physician Assistants (AAPA), every state chapter of the AAPA, the National Commission on Certification of Physician Assistants (NCCPA), CASPA applications, and the Physician Assistant Education Association (PAEA), just to name a few. Think about the cost, alone, to change every piece of literature?

All this information would change how this prompt could be answered. I provided a list of examples for illustrative purposes only, so that you can see the talking points you may want to use during the body of your answer. In the actual MMI, only focus on bringing up missing information that you believe would alter your answer, rather than a laundry list.

For example, how would physicians react to a name change? The name "physician associate" was used initially when the profession began; however, physicians weren't too fond of that name (and were perhaps threatened), and it was changed to "physician assistant." Would the same situation occur if the name is changed now?

Ask the interviewer, "Can you provide me with any more information about any of these questions I just raised?" In many cases the interviewer will not provide additional information. If she doesn't, quickly state your assumptions so you can move forward efficiently with your response.

EXAMPLE

"Assuming physicians will no longer protest the name change…"

Let's look at the prompt again and consider the issues from multiple perspectives. This information will provide the body of your response.

It has been long debated in the PA profession whether to change the name of the profession from *physician assistant* to *physician associate*. Many PAs feel that the word *assistant* does not accurately reflect the advanced training and abilities that PAs have, and they feel patients mistake them as medical assistants. If you frequent the PA Forum (physicianassistantforum.com), you will find a variety of comments on this topic. Most favor changing the name to Physician Associate. In a small poll posted on Inside PA Training's website (mypatraining.com,) 507 participants voted on this topic. Here are the results:

▶ 360 participants (71.01%) voted to change the name to "physician associate"

- 79 participants (15.58%) voted not to change the name
- 60 participants (13.41%) voted to change the name, but not to "physician associate"

If you had the tie-breaking vote on choosing to keep the name or change the name, how would you vote and why? Would you change the name to physician associate? Would you change the name to something else? Would you keep the name as it is? Who should be considered before making your decision?

The Actors, the Missing Information, and the Issues

EXAMPLE FROM MULTIPLE PERSPECTIVES

- Vote to change the name of the profession.

A vote would have to be taken at the national level, including as many PAs as possible. The sample poll mentioned in the prompt only includes 507 voters, which is not large enough to rely upon, and certainly doesn't capture the opinions of the entire PA profession. Using a larger voting pool may yield a different result.

I would also consider whether PA students and PA faculty members would be included in the vote.

I would also be very interested as to the *reason* the voters would choose to change the name. Is it an ego issue, or is the reason related to more principal issues?

- Vote to change the name to something different.

I think there should also be a discussion amongst PAs about other options for a name change. Some PAs have suggested simply using "PA" as the name of the profession. However, I feel that it is still important to poll PAs about changing the name, and just as important, what would be the *reason* for the name change. If the profession voted to change the name of the profession, the reasons for the change should also be considered.

▶ Consider the public.

The physician assistant profession enjoys high patient satisfaction ratings, right up there with nurse practitioners and physicians. PAs enjoy higher-than-average salaries than their college graduate colleagues, and the BLS continues to rank the future of the PA profession as very promising. PAs have also done a remarkable job of educating patients over many years as to what their role is and how they fit into the healthcare system. Would a name change set the profession back by causing more confusion with patients? Would PAs have to spend years reeducating patients? Would a name change provide the profession with even higher satisfaction ratings? I believe having patient focus groups might provide more clarity to these questions.

What would be the benefit? Higher salaries? An even better satisfaction rating? A higher score by BLS? Better patient care? I think there may be more questions than answers.

▶ Consider physicians' response to a name change.

Early in the profession, physicians were the ones responsible for the profession changing its name from "physician associate" to "physician assistant." They felt threatened by the name "physician associate" and thought the name may be confusing to patients. It might be a clever idea to include physicians in the process if a name change were to take place. Taking this step could avoid the same dilemma in the future if the name is changed.

▶ Consider the logistics of a name change.

Once a name change occurs, there will be a financial burden on the profession to change the name on every website, administrative agency, and PA program. All the current literature relating to the physician assistant profession would have to be discarded and redone to reflect the new name, whether it be physician associate or some other name. The costs and logistics of doing so would have to justify the name change. There would have to be a thorough investigation on the financial component to weigh the pros and cons of the name change.

▶ My experience.

NOTE: *As mentioned previously, it's a good idea to include a personal experience in your answer. Using a personal example shows that you have experience with these issues and you really understand the issues brought up in the prompt, and the most effective way of dealing with them.*

Concluding Your Response

Hopefully you feel a little more comfortable now that you have a blueprint for answering MMI questions, and the ability to show how the actors and stakeholders are affected. The next step in the process is the conclusion of your response.

At the end of your response, you'll want to make sure that you end effectively. You've already stated that the prompt is missing some information that could change your answer, and you've stated the relative assumptions that will impact your response.

Now arrive at your conclusion that makes sense given the analysis you've already provided:

- ▸ Relate the prompt to healthcare.
- ▸ Use a personal example.
- ▸ Extend the dialogue.
- ▸ Summarize.

A possible conclusion to this prompt could be:

Changing the name of the PA profession from "physician assistant" to "physician associate" has been up for debate for several years. The PA profession celebrated fifty years in October 2017. The profession is also consistently ranked as one of the top ten professions by the Bureau of Labor Statistics. One option to consider is, "If it isn't broken, why fix it?"

However, if a name change is going to be contemplated, there would need to be a vote at the national level amongst as many PAs as possible. I think the AAPA would probably need to set up a task force to consider the impact of changing the name. It will also be important when considering a name change to ask *why* to change the name? What is the reason for a name change now?

Additionally, before the name is changed, there would have to be a consensus amongst PAs and a decision on what the profession's name would be changed to. After a vote, it may be changed to something other than physician associate. Perhaps simply "PA" would be an appropriate name? After all, many nurse practitioners address themselves as APRNs. Patients are already familiar and comfortable with the name PA, and the word "assistant," which seems to be of concern to so many current PAs, would be eliminated.

The public (patients) should also be considered in this decision. Over the past fifty years, PAs have done a very effective job educating the public about the PA profession, and the profession currently enjoys a high satisfaction rating equal to NPs and physicians. PAs should consider whether a name change will be confusing to patients, who will have to be reeducated concerning the name change. Will a name change upset patients? I would hope patients would be included in the AAPA focus group before deciding.

PAs also needs to consider that a name change to "physician associate" was rejected by physicians in the early years of the profession. Therefore, I believe any focus groups should also include physicians. The debate about a name change has been solely discussed amongst PAs, to date. It would be beneficial to get the physicians' point of view and have a preliminary opinion from physician focus groups on the name change before investing the resources to choose and change the name. I'm glad this question/prompt was included in the interview. I have some experience working on focus groups while I was a patient relations representative in a large city hospital. We often invited patients to participate in the focus groups to see what the hospital was doing right, and areas where the hospital could improve. I found it very interesting how our preconceived notions about how we were performing, often weren't reflected in the patients' responses.

In summary, there is a lot of missing information and actors involved, which makes it difficult for me to give a direct answer. There seem to be more questions than answers. I would be in favor of a name change if Full Practice Authority and Responsibility were granted to PAs. I would vote to change the name to physician associate, but I would also be open to other names that haven't been considered yet.

To conclude your answer to the prompt, you will need a strong ending. Provide a clear summary of your talking points. This is a good way to end effectively as it reinforces the strongest ideas from your response and leaves a positive lasting impression. Take a moment to decide how you would conclude. Relate this prompt to yourself and summarize the talking points.

The next thing you will want to do after concluding your response is to ask follow-up questions. Asking follow-up questions allows you to extend the dialogue with the interviewer. By extending the dialogue you can use the skills you learned from Chapter 8, Winning Through High Impact Communication, to come across as likeable, credible, and trustworthy.

Because MMI's tend to be very stressful, do your best to make a positive impression on your interviewer:

- ▸ Smile
- ▸ Make eye contact
- ▸ Use open gestures
- ▸ Breathe!

Additionally, to keep your anxiety to a minimum, don't forget to use the SHIELD technique (presented on page 186), either before you enter the room, or at each break. Utilizing this technique will lower your adrenaline levels and keep you out of the "fight or flight mode."

Finally, don't forget that in addition to question-type prompts, you may also have a role-playing scenario, or you may have to label the structures on a body part, or even teach someone how to perform a specific task.

Follow-Up Questions

The remainder of your time should be aimed at allowing for follow-up questions, as applicable. Remember, it is advantageous to turn a monologue into a dialogue. Answering follow-up questions allows the interviewer to speak and get clarification on any number of issues you've raised. A follow-up question is also an opportunity for you to show your ability to adapt quickly.

Review

Outside the Room

Take the two or three minutes allowed to read the prompt, reread the prompt, and plan a response based on the skills the prompt is trying to elicit. Develop bullet points to help you structure your answer. Consider the actors, issues, missing information, and multiple perspectives.

Inside the Room

Start out by giving a summary of the prompt, and ask, "Do I have this right?" This will ensure that you and the interviewer are on the same page.

Consider the most important parts of the prompt, then analyze and present those parts. These will be the bullet points you developed outside of the room. Consider who the actors are, if there is any missing information, and consider the prompt from multiple perspectives.

Finally, end effectively by arriving at a conclusion and supporting your argument through personal examples. Extend the dialogue by examining follow-up opportunities.

Then, allow time to respond to any of the interviewer's follow-up questions.

Remember: In the traditional chapters I stressed the importance of Qualities. Be sure to incorporate as many of your Qualities as possible into your answer.

Final Thoughts

I hope I have demystified the MMI for you. It is a challenging interview format, and those who are best prepared will score highest.

Prior to attending a MMI format interview, try finding out the duration of the stations, both inside and outside of the room, the number of stations, the number of rest breaks, the length of the entire interview, and if you will be allowed to take notes and use them inside the room.

Don't be afraid to call the program directly to find out this information. You can also check the program's website, Facebook page, or even go on the PA Forum (physicianassistantforum.com) and check for any information provided from student or other applicants who may have interviewed at the program.

Although most applicants view the MMI interview favorably, a considerable number of applicants have shared with me that their experience was concerning. There are four typical areas of concerns my coaching applicants have reported back to me:

1. **Lack of Control.** Many applicants feel as though they didn't have enough time to talk about the things like work experience, personal interests, and Qualities. They also feel that five or six minutes was not enough time to fully complete their thoughts.

2. **Anxiety and Nervousness.** Some applicants report being so nervous and anxious that they could not think clearly and were unable to communicate their thoughts in a cohesive manner.

3. **Inability to Move Past Inferior Performance on a Previous Station.** If an applicant felt she did not do well on the previous station, she was unable to let go and stay in the moment at subsequent stations.

4. **Approach Taken by Interviewers.** Some applicants report being intimidated by the aggressiveness of one or more of the interviewers.

Remember, the only way to provide effective answers to MMI prompts is to practice. The MMI is not an interview where you can "wing it."

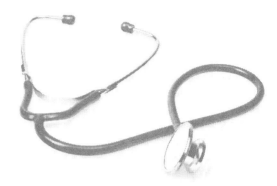

CHAPTER 8

Winning Through High-Impact Communication

In this chapter, I'm going to teach you a secret that really separates the Perfect Applicants from the vanilla applicants at the interview. You may be surprised to know that an applicant can answer all the interview questions perfectly, yet still not get accepted because they fail to understand the following secret:

The admissions committee selects candidates based on an emotional decision and justifies that decision with the facts.

Once you leave the interview room, the interviewer(s) won't pull out a chalk board and write down facts such as your GPA, GRE, how many questions you answered correctly, and how many questions you answered incorrectly. They don't tally up the numbers and decide based on some sort of scoring system. Based on my experience on the admissions committee, the typical response when you leave the room is either "I really like her" or "I don't like her." Your score is based on your likeability and the connection you made with the committee.

This chapter will teach you how to maximize your communication skills and use them to your advantage during your interview.

High-Impact Communication

Winning Through High-Impact Communication

Okay, I may date myself with some of the examples in this section. You may not be fully aware of who some of the players are, but it really doesn't matter. I just want you to grasp the point I'm trying to make, versus the names of the people I mention to make my point.

Funk and Wagnall's dictionary defines charisma as *extraordinary personal power or charm*. To some it comes naturally, but often it must be learned. Charisma is a result of a series of behaviors through which someone has a powerful and positive impact on others. In this chapter, we will teach you how to develop your own personal charisma to build a bridge to credibility and trust.

Barack Obama, Bill Clinton, and Malala Yousafzai all have charisma. They move beyond facts, figures, and fancy jargon and seek a connection when they speak. For you to "connect" with your interviewer, you will need to learn what these effective communicators already know.

Malala Yousafzai gained international attention and acclaim when she, as a young teenager, advocated for the rights of young women to attend school in her Taliban-controlled town, resulting in her attempted assassination. She survived, and even from her hospital bed, continued to speak out against the discrimination and violence. Even before that, at eleven years old, she worked with the BBC to share information on the occupation's impact on daily life in the region. Her words reached millions as she began to travel and share her story, from the UN to Harvard University. Her book was an overnight bestseller. At age seventeen, she became the youngest ever Nobel Peace Prize winner, and continues to advocate for human rights against tyrannical regimes all over the world.

Why did the world connect with Malala? She demonstrated strength, integrity, and perseverance. On top of that, she knows how to communicate, effectively, persuasively, and above all, believably. She not only reaches the part of our minds that seek out stories of human achievement over adversity, but also the part that reacts to openness, feeling, enthusiasm, and energy—the primitive brain.

The Emotional Gatekeeper (The Primitive Brain)

In all the presidential elections since 1960, those who won reached our primitive brain; those who lost didn't. How can you increase your chances of getting accepted to PA school? By reaching the primitive brain. It is the secret of believability! It's real, physical, and powerful. Neglect it, ignore it, fail to harness its power, and you'll likely fail to connect with your interviewer.

In 2012, former Massachussetts Governor Mitt Romney, in his race for the White House, tasted defeat because he failed to connect with the people on a personal level. Bill Walsh (Hall of Fame football coach) has eluded broadcasting fame because he can't connect. Dan Rather, the anchor for CBS News from the 1980s into the early 2000s, is the reason CBS lagged ABC and NBC with respect to the ratings. These people don't know the secret that I will share with you later.

"But I'm not in the public eye," you might say. Not exactly. As PAs, we're *all* in the public eye. The ability to communicate effectively is the single most important skill you need to succeed as a PA.

So, why do people miss the boat on effective communication? They fail to realize that communication is a contact sport.

Communication Is a Contact Sport

Barack Obama ran against John McCain for president in 2008. Obama was a junior senator in his first term, and McCain was a senior senator, having served in the senate since 1987. In his prior life, Barack Obama was a community organizer in Chicago. John McCain was a former POW and war hero. On paper, John McCain was clearly the stronger candidate. So why did he lose so convincingly? Barack Obama has charisma!

Barack Obama is a master communicator. He understands how to connect with an audience, verbally, vocally, and visually. He smiles and uses open gestures which make him likeable and trustworthy.

John McCain, on the other hand, rarely smiles, appears to be very "stiff" when speaking, and doesn't use open gestures. John McCain lacks charisma.

Now let's look at Bill Walsh, the renowned ex-professional football coach. He won Super Bowls with the San Francisco 49ers, he is technically precise, experienced, good looking, and considered a football genius. This is the perfect combination for a career as a successful broadcaster, right?

The problem is that Bill Walsh has a nasal voice, he rarely smiles, and most of all, he fails to recognize that communication is a contact sport. He went from a short stint in the broadcast booth to coaching college football, and back to the 49ers as a consultant.

In contrast, there's John Madden. He quit as the Oakland Raiders football coach, has a face only a mother can love, and he's extremely difficult to schedule because he won't fly. Yet John Madden had million-dollar contracts with the Fox TV network, Miller Lite, and Ace hardware—why? He has charisma, credibility, and trust. He's honest, natural, and most of all, he's believable.

Creating Emotional Impact

You must sell yourself to create emotional impact.

While preparing for one of my seminars many years ago, I received an email from a person on the staff of a PA program in the southern United States. He wanted to "join the team" and help me out with my upcoming seminars. I wrote back thanking him for his interest but telling him that I was not looking to hire anyone at this point. I never heard from him again.

A week later, I received a telephone call from another person wanting to come aboard and help me out. This person, Chris, told me that he had seven years' experience on one of the local PA program's admissions committees. He sold me on the idea that he would truly be an asset to our program. He understood the power of a living résumé versus words on a computer screen. Chris understood that he was selling himself and his Qualities, so I offered him a position.

What are you selling?

Some people become uncomfortable when I mention the word "selling." But we all sell ourselves every day. We sell our ideas, our concepts, our Qualities, and our reasons why the admissions committee should select us over other highly qualified candidates.

The Secret

If you buy into the fact that we are all selling *something*, then you must understand this crucial point mentioned earlier. It's worth repeating here; **The admissions committee selects candidates based on emotion, and justifies its decision with the facts.** That's the secret in this book that many applicants I've interviewed don't understand. But it's a principal that will help you get accepted!

As mentioned earlier, after a candidate walks out of the interview room, the committee doesn't sit down with a yellow pad, draw a line down the center, and list the positives and negatives with respect to your presentation. Rather, the decision to accept you or not is more influenced by emotional factors versus rational factors alone. If they like you on an emotional level, they'll justify giving you a higher score by commenting on your GPA, test scores, experience, or whatever will work to support this emotionally based decision. If the committee doesn't like you on an emotional level, you can have a 4.0 GPA, top GRE scores, and ten years of hands-on medical experience as an EMT, and still not win their support.

Statistics are Cold and Cerebral

In 1960 JFK trailed Nixon at the polls 53% to 47%. By election day, however, JFK shot ahead—why? TV. Nixon won on radio with debating points, but JFK won the television audience on emotion. Nixon tried to appeal based on facts, records, and statistics. "I attended 217 meetings with the National Security Council. I attended 63 cabinet meetings and presided over 19 of them. I visited 54 countries...," etc. The problem is that statistics are cold and cerebral, and so too, the nation concluded, was Richard M. Nixon. The cold war-weary voters found Kennedy reassuring when compared to Nixon. JFK understood how to make emotional contact with his audience.

Are you what I call a "paper star?" You look great on paper and feel that your GPA and experience alone should get you into PA school? That's not how it works. PAs must communicate daily with their patients, supervising physicians, and families. If you are too cold and cerebral, you won't connect in this arena, either. Therefore, any PA program worth applying to will interview candidates, and not select them based solely on their GPA or GRE scores.

Some programs have an absolute criterion for GRE scores to be considered for an interview. I believe these programs are doing themselves, and the PA profession, a disservice by prioritizing statistics as a deciding factor in whether an applicant will make a good PA.

Some applicants tend to intuitively grasp what it means to communicate effectively and emotionally. The rest of us must learn it and work at it. This chapter will provide the techniques that you need to create an emotional connection with others.

These techniques, which will improve your eye contact, energetic delivery, and the ability to think on your feet, to name just a few, will enhance your personal impact in communicating with the admissions committee.

Three Truths

Personal impact is power. Power to achieve whatever you want in your personal life and career. The secret to obtaining personal power is based on three fundamental truths.

▶ **Truth #1: The spoken word is the polar opposite of the written word.**

The written word is linear, single channel communication that goes directly to the cerebral cortex, a highly developed reasoning and analytical portion of the brain. The spoken word is multichannel and includes a kaleidoscope of nonverbal cues such as posture, eye contact, energy, volume, intonation, and much more. Spoken communication carries energy, feeling, passion, and goes directly to the emotional center of the brain—the primitive brain.

The facts are clear: If all you want to do is transfer information, put it in writing. But if you need to motivate, persuade, and influence people, say it with impact.

▶ **Truth #2:** What you say must be believed to have impact.

No message, no matter how eloquently stated, brilliantly defended, or painstakingly documented, can penetrate a wall of distrust, apprehension, and indifference. For your message to be believed, *you* must be believed.

At Yale, we interviewed a young woman who was an accomplished off-Broadway actress. She presented us with a very creative and off-beat resume. At the bottom right-hand corner of the resume, below all her credits as an actress, she typed, "Special Talents: I can tie a cherry stem into a knot with my tongue." I still speak about this résumé twenty years later.

This young woman lost her credibility with me before she even walked into the room. One of my colleagues was even more offended. She asked the applicant during her interview: "Tell us about your most memorable patient." The actress started to cry and describe an illness that her mother had overcome. My colleague asked her at this point, "How do we know you're not acting now?" Ouch! The applicant was stunned and she knew the interview was over, and so were her chances of getting accepted to Yale. She had set herself up for failure before she entered the room to interview.

Our "gut-feeling" on whether we like and believe someone or not is based on emotion versus logic and fact. Does your voice crack? Do your eyes flicker and dart? Is your posture wrong? Do your hands fidget? Are you *acting*?

▶ **Truth #3:** Believability is determined at the preconscious level.

Perhaps this is the most important truth. Where does believability come from? You can't build believability out of a mountain of facts and figures. You can't even build it out of a stack of eloquently crafted words. Authoritative credentials, a title, or a letter of recommendation from a big-shot may give you some credibility and get you to the interview, but you still must be believable to get accepted into PA school.

There are five rules to make yourself more believable:

1. Make eye contact.
2. Smile.
3. Use open gestures.
4. Use a firm handshake.
5. Have good posture and a strong voice.

Interviewers Are Bombarded with Visual Stimuli that Register at the Preconscious Level

The moment we walk into an interview, we begin giving off a series of verbal and nonverbal cues. Do we stand tall when we walk into the room, or are we slumped over? Do we give a firm handshake, or do we have a limp handshake with sweaty palms? During the interview, do we refer to our patients as "arms and legs," or do we refer to them by name? Do we refer to nurses in a derogatory manner, or do we give them the respect they deserve?

An enormous amount of communication is taking place as these thousands of multichannel impressions are carried to your brain. Most of these impressions register at the preconscious level. Because of these impressions, the brain forms a continuous stream of emotional judgments and assessments. Do I trust this person? Is she honest, evasive, friendly, or threatening? Is he interesting, boring, warm, cold, anxious? Is she confident, insecure, appear to be hiding something?

The emotional judgment that is formed in your preconscious mind about the speaker determines whether you will tune in to the message or tune it out. If you don't believe in someone at the emotional level, little of what they say will get through.

Discovering Primitive Brain Power

The $25 Million Dollar Lesson

In 1989, Deborah Norville was hired by NBC to co-host the Today show with Jane Pauley. This was a classic case of "If it isn't broke, don't fix it!" Norville was intelligent and had journalistic credibility, but she also seemed unapproachable and cold. Jane Pauley became lost in the shuffle, and in December 1989 a misty-eyed Pauley said goodbye to the *Today* show.

When Pauley left, she took the dynamic chemistry with her. Don't worry about Jane, however; she came back strong. The uncertain future wasn't Jane Pauley's, but the *Today* show itself. With Jane, the show enjoyed a 4.4 rating and a 21 share. In the first quarter of 1990 the show dropped to a 3.5 rating and an 18 share. The total cost to NBC was $25 million. Heads rolled, and people were fired.

What did Jane Pauley have that Deborah Norville didn't? In a word, warmth. An open smile with a touch of wit behind it. An honest sense of humor, a delightful sparkle. A bit of the "girl next door" quality. Deborah Norville offered a sexy brand of competence and the cool, unapproachable beauty of a prom queen. NBC seriously miscalculated thinking that Americans would prefer to wake and have breakfast with the prom queen rather than the girl next door.

Eventually, NBC saw the light and hired Katie Couric. Soon after, the ratings soared again—why? She has that "girl next door" quality too. Glamour is not the key ingredient. Beauty and competence are not enough. You must learn to connect with your audience.

How Does the Brain Work?

Anatomy & Physiology 101

All communication must pass the gatekeeper: the primitive brain. Will our message get through or will it be blocked? Do you represent friend or foe? Do you know how to befriend the gatekeeper?

Contrary to what you've probably been taught, effective communication is only partly concerned with our intellectual human brain, or neocortex (new brain). Before we can communicate effectively with our listener's new brain, we must consider a hidden and generally unrecognized part of ourselves. The primitive brain, although it is hidden from our conscious, is real, it is physical, and it is extremely powerful.

If the top brass at NBC understood how this worked, Jane Pauley would not have been fired, and NBC would have been millions richer. If John McCain understood how the primitive brain works, he might have gone to the White House. It's not mysterious, but it is new. The last several years have increased our knowledge of the brain tenfold. We can now analyze why certain people behave in certain ways to make that all-important connection in their communication. We call it "demystifying charisma."

Very simply, our brain is composed of the first brain, or primitive brain, and the new brain (neocortex) or cerebral cortex. The cerebral cortex is the thinking, rational portion of our brain. The new brain is three to four million years old. The "left" side of our new brain deals with learning, math, and writing. The "right" side of our new brain deals with art and inspiration. The new brain, however, pales in significance to the primitive, first brain.

The primitive brain is the irrational, emotional part of our brain: the gatekeeper. The primitive brain is two hundred to five hundred million years old and is composed mainly of the limbic system. The primitive brain is the seat of human emotion. Your task at your interview is to reach the primitive brain first.

The Goal: Get to the New Brain via the Primitive Brain

When people communicate with the spoken word, they almost invariably aim the message at the new brain and completely overlook the primitive brain. That's why even competent and intellectual people can fail to effectively communicate a message to their audiences. This is not to say the new brain is unimportant; on the contrary, our goal is really to get our message to the new brain because that's the decision-making part. But to reach the new brain, our message must first pass the primitive brain—the emotional gatekeeper. If we ignore this, our message will be distorted or diminished, or it may not get through at all.

It's the listener's primitive brain that decides whether to trust you. It's the primitive brain that decides whether a person represents comfort and safety or anxiety and menace. The key to understanding the primitive brain is recognizing that its sole purpose is survival. It quickly analyzes all incoming data and asks the questions: "Is the situation safe? Friend or foe?" You must convince your listener's primitive brain that you are likeable—that you represent warmth, comfort, and safety.

Try this exercise. Take your right hand and make a fist with your right thumb pointing at your face. Now take your left hand, palm facing down, and wrap it around your right fist. This model represents your brain. Your left hand represents your cerebral cortex, the thinking, decision-making portion of the brain. Your right fist is your primitive brain and includes the limbic system. From here arises memory, pain, pleasure, and the ability to balance the extremes of emotion.

Now, you ask, what is the thumb doing pointing at my face? Here is one of the most important new discoveries: the connection between the sensory organs and the primitive brain. Your right thumbnail represents your eyes. The thumb represents the nerve pathways from your eyes to the primitive brain. All your sensory input—visual from the eyes, sound from the ears, taste, touch, and smell—goes to the primitive brain *first*.

Now that you understand the physiological relationship between the primitive brain and the new brain, let's review and examine some of the differences between these two brain systems. As mentioned, the primitive brain is two hundred to five hundred million years old;

the new brain is three to four million years old. The primitive brain is instinctual and primitive; the new brain is intellectual and advanced. The primitive brain is emotional; the new brain is rational. Most importantly, perhaps, is that the primitive brain is unconscious, and the new brain is conscious.

Today, scientists are rejecting the notion of man being simply a thinking machine, and are beginning to see human beings instead as biological organisms whose survival depends on constant interaction with the environment. Emotions contain the "wisdom of the ages," as one expert put it.

The Limbic System

The limbic system, embedded deep in the brain, encompasses all sensory input. For example, have you ever had an immediate and strong emotional response when you first caught the smell of baking bread in the oven, or the scent of leaves on a crisp autumn day, or the salty sea air blowing in from the ocean? Although your new brain will figure out where the feeling comes from, often lodged deep within your memory, it was the olfactory bulbs of the limbic system that gave that emotional reaction even before you became conscious of why. Smell and the sound of music both appear to be the language of the primitive brain, often triggering an immediate emotional response.

When I sold real estate, I was trained to place a teaspoon of vanilla in a small pan into a hot oven in the home I was showing. Why? The vanilla gave the scent of baking bread. This powerful scent has a strong reaction on the buyer's olfactory bulbs that makes them feel like they are in a home rather than a regular building.

Scientists now believe that the limbic system is not only the center of emotional stimulus, but it is the main switching station for all sensory input. It determines what sensory input is passed on to the new brain for analysis and decision-making, and what input is filtered out and ignored.

Leslie Hart is the brain expert who wrote *How the Brain Works*. He said this about gatekeeping: "Much evidence now indicates that the limbic area in the first brain is the main switch in determining what sensory input will go to the neocortex and what decisions will be accepted from it."

All the signals that you give off when you speak, including your mannerisms, gestures, eye contact, inflection, and other nonverbal cues, pass through the limbic system for processing. Now, if these nonverbal cues convince the limbic system that you are friendly, the message gets a clear channel to the decision-making processes in the new brain. But, if these cues suggest that you are an uncomfortable, threatening presence, the limbic system will alter or block your message.

So, if we are energetic, enthusiastic, and believable, our words will actually be given more impact and energy by the listener's primitive brain before they are switched to the new brain. But if we appear boring, anxious, and insecure, our words may not even reach their destination. Instead, our message will be discolored or even tuned out at the switching station by a lack of believability.

How, then, do we make friends with the gatekeeper so that our message can get through? How do we become primitive brain friendly? By being natural, and by learning to use natural energy, enthusiasm, and gestures—all the multichannel, nonverbal cues that enable us to make emotional contact with our listeners. Emotion is the key to making communication memorable. To persuade others and achieve your goals, you must understand the primitive brain concept. It all depends on you.

Getting to Trust

How do we use our natural self to reach the primitive brains of our listeners? You've got to be believed to be heard. When dealing with people, trust and believability are synonymous. You can't have one without the other. To communicate effectively with others, you must be trusted. And to win their trust, you must be believable. Belief is a primitive brain function; it's acceptance on faith, it's emotionally based, and it bypasses the intellect. Your primitive brain speaks the language of behavior.

While our new brain sifts our communication for content, data, and facts, our primitive brain looks for nuances of behavior. Does the voice quiver, or does it project authority? Do your eyes flicker hesitantly or gaze unflinchingly? Is your posture confident or diffident? This is the language of the primitive brain, the language of trust.

Who we trust and why is often learned as a baby. One day my son, Eddie, and I were at the airport in Hartford, Connecticut. We were on our way to Orlando, Florida to present a seminar. While sitting in the chairs by our gate, we noticed a toddler walking over to us with a smile from ear to ear. She was cooing and drooling and having a grand old time. My son and I both played peek-a-boo with her and she shrieked with laughter. She then walked over to another passenger waiting for his plane, with that same big smile. He gave her a serious look that said, "I'm not interested little girl; go away, you're bothering me." The little girl's eyes opened wide, and she immediately began to pout and cry. She ran from that man knowing instinctively he represented trouble; he was not safe.

You can't communicate with a baby using words; rather, we must use facial expressions, energy, and sound. The baby responds with the same set of verbal cues. The smile is the language of primitive brain communication. Even a baby knows that a person who doesn't smile lacks warmth and safety. We learn early that the people we should trust are those who smile. To communicate effectively, we must relearn the language of trust.

Did you ever meet someone and instantly like or dislike her, but you didn't know why? When you meet someone for the first time, your primitive brain receives thousands of nonverbal cues that are registered at the preconscious level. Your intuition comes from this; you form an almost immediate impression of that person. You form an impression that is detailed and often richly colored with emotion.

Most candidates approach the PA school interview as though it's all new-brain communication. Their arguments are logic and reason: GPA scores, GRE scores, medical experience, and providing strong answers to interview questions. The fact is, an equal or greater part of all human communication is primitive-brain intuition. When you leave the interview, the committee uses words like, "I liked him," or "I don't trust her," or "There's something about her that I really like."

Some people can naturally do this without understanding how it works. The candidate who speaks the language of the primitive brain, the language of trust, is the candidate most likely to be believed and accepted. That language communicates very rapidly and effectively.

The Likeability Factor

In 1984, President Reagan ran for re-election against Walter Mondale. A Gallup Poll looked at three areas with respect to the candidates: issues, part affiliation, and likeability. On the issues, the candidates were considered to be dead even. However, The Democrat (Mondale) clearly had the edge when it came to party affiliation. With respect to likeability, though, Reagan had the edge and won the election. It was the personality factor that dominated.

As applicants, we pride ourselves on our great GPA, our medical experience, and our GRE scores. But when it's time to interview, it's your likeability that determines whether you receive an acceptance letter or a rejection letter. And as soon as you walk into that interview room, it's the visual connection that sets the beginning of trust and credibility.

The Eye Factor

The eye is the only sensory organ that contains brain cells. Memory experts invariably link the objects they remember to a visual image. Research shows that it's the visual image that makes the greatest impact in communication.

The spoken message is made up of only three components:

▸ The **verbal**
▸ The **vocal**
▸ The **visual**

In the 1960s, a prominent professor at UCLA, Albert Mehrabian, pioneered a landmark study on the relationship of the three components of the spoken word. He measured the effect of each on the believability of the spoken message. The **verbal** message, or the actual words we use, are what most people mistakenly concentrate on. In fact, this is the smallest part of the spoken message. The **vocal** component is made up of the intonation, projection, and resonance of your spoken message. It is the **visual** message, however—the emotion and expression of your body and face as you speak—that carries the most weight.

Mehrabian also found that the degree of consistency or inconsistency between these three key elements determines the believability of your message. The more these three factors harmonize, the more believable you are as a candidate. If your verbal message is not in harmony with your body language, you send a mixed signal to the primitive brain. Your message may or may not get through to the decision-making new brain. Mehrabian quantified the three components of the spoken message as follows:

▸ **Verbal** = 7%
▸ **Voice** = 38%
▸ **Visual** = 55%

In other words, what you see is what you get. If you come into the interview room yawning or inappropriately dressed, nothing you do or say will help you. The interviewer's primitive brain has already decided your fate.

How Do We Enhance versus Inhibit Our Message?

The first way we enhance our communication is with eye contact. This is the number one skill to develop; it's primitive brain to primitive brain. The three rules and exercises for maintaining eye contact are as follows:

Rules

1. Use involvement rather than intimacy or intimidation.
2. Count to five (involvement) then look away.
3. Don't dart your eyes, as this represents a lack of confidence.

Exercises

1. **Use video feedback.** Tape yourself speaking with someone and watch your use or violation of the three rules.
2. **Practice one-on-one.** Have a conversation with someone you trust and ask them for direct feedback with respect to these rules.
3. **Practice with a paper audience.** Place sticky notes with happy faces drawn on them onto a chair. Practice counting to five and looking away after five seconds before shifting your gaze to the next sticky note (person).

The next way to enhance our message is with posture and movement. A good posture commands attention, and movement shows confidence. Walk into the room standing tall. Don't slump. When you speak to your interviewer, don't be afraid to add movement to your message. You don't have to wave your hands all over the place, but use open gestures to better come across as a friendly, open person.

Rules

1. Stand tall.
2. Watch your lower body; don't lean back on one hip or rock back and forth.

3. Get in the "ready position." Lean slightly forward if you're sitting, or onto the balls of your feet if you're standing.
4. Move; show that you're excited, enthusiastic, and confident.

Exercises

1. **Walk away from the wall.** Stand with your back against a wall, heels pressed against the wall along with your head, neck, and shoulders. Try to push the small of your back into the wall. Now simply walk away from the wall and feel how upright and correct your posture is. Try to shake off this posture; you can't. Practice this daily so that when you walk into the interview room, you'll command attention.

2. **Use the ready position.** Remember, if you're standing, push up slightly on the balls of your feet. If you are sitting, lean slightly forward to your interviewer(s).

3. **Use a paper audience.**

The third way to enhance your message is with dress and appearance. You only get two seconds to make your initial impression on your interviewer. If you blow it, it may take over thirty minutes to recover, and most candidates only get twenty minutes, maximum. So, it is critical to make a good first impression.

When you are dressed up for an interview, only 10% of your skin is exposed. Please be sure that this 10% is clean, free of extravagant jewelry, trimmed, combed, and smells good (no tobacco smell).

Rules

1. Be appropriate; "When in Rome..."
2. Be conservative. When in doubt, dress up.
3. Men, always button your jacket.
4. Don't overkill perfume or cologne, and certainly don't smoke on the day of your interview.
5. Always bring a small mirror and check your face, teeth, and hair before interviewing.

Exercises

1. **Get feedback.** Ask friends and relatives how well you present yourself.
2. **Be observant.** Look at some fashion magazines. Find a style in which you are comfortable.

The final way to enhance your message is with gestures and your smile. Do you speak with conviction, enthusiasm, and passion? Are you friendly or stuffy? Do you speak with open gestures and a warm smile, or are you a "fig-leaf flasher," with your hands always going back and forth covering your groin? Remember, openness equals likeability.

Rules

1. Identify nervous gestures and stop them.
2. "Lift your apples"—smile. Make believe you have apples on your cheekbones and try to lift them up to your forehead.
3. Feel your smile.
4. Caution: Phony smiles don't work.

Exercises

1. **Imitate someone you feel is an effective communicator and play the part with gusto.** Get used to using open gestures and expressions.
2. **Be natural.** Incorporate some of these gestures into your daily communication.

The eye factor rules. The language of the primitive brain is visual language.

The Energy Factor

Energy is the fuel that drives the car to success. You don't want to run out of gas when you're halfway up the hill. Think back to the last morning when you woke up and felt like you could conquer the world; this was a powerful space to be in. That is where you need to be on interview day—"in the zone," if you will. This next section will focus on ways to unlock your inner energy and present yourself in the best light to the admissions committee.

Voice and Vocal Variety

Try to use positive intonation and inflection in your voice. Speaking in a monotone can be deadly and put your listener to sleep. Observe and practice the following rules and exercises to add a bit of personal style to your voice. Follow these five rules:

1. Make your voice naturally authoritative by speaking from the diaphragm.
2. Put your voice on a roller coaster; practice reading from magazines using intonation and inflection.
3. Be aware of your telephone voice; it represents 84% of the emotional impact when people can't see you.
4. Smile while you speak on the telephone. People can feel your smile when you speak.
5. Put your real feelings into your voice.

To improve your voice and vocal variety, practice these three exercises:

1. **Breathe from the diaphragm.** Take in a deep breath from your nose and let it out slowly, stopping to feel the pressure on your diaphragm. This is where a strong voice originates.
2. **Project your voice.** Try speaking in a normal voice first, then project your voice to reach the back of the room. Try to find the right depth to your voice without straining your vocal chords.
3. **Practice varying your pitch and pace.** Read from magazines.

Words and Non-Words

Energize with words:

1. Build your vocabulary, especially with synonyms. Instead of "give," use "endow." Instead of "follower," use "disciple." Instead of "cloudy," use "obscure." However, make sure you know the exact definition of the synonyms so that you use them correctly!
2. Paint word pictures. Use motion and emotion with metaphors.
3. Beware of jargon, especially medical jargon. Use "operating room," instead of "OR," and use "physician" rather than "Doc."
4. Avoid meaningless non-words like "ahh," "uhm," "so," "well." "you know," and "like." Replace these non-words with a powerful *pause*. A properly timed pause adds drama, energy, and power to your message. Every time you catch yourself getting ready to use a non-word, pause instead. This takes a little practice, but will enhance your message tremendously.

Listener Involvement

Humans communicate; books dispense information. Try using these key techniques to add an extra punch to your communication.

1. Use a strong opening. Make it visual and energetic by including pauses, action and motion, joy, and laughter.
2. Maintain eye contact. When you enter the room for a group interview, survey your listeners for three to five seconds, gauge, and adjust. Be sure to include all of the interviewers with eye contact.
3. Lean toward your listeners.
4. Create interest by maintaining eye contact and having high energy.

Humor

"I will not make age an issue in this campaign. I am not going to exploit, for political purposes, my opponent's youth and inexperience." These words, spoken during a presidential debate in 1984, changed the entire campaign for Ronald Reagan. Reagan knew that he was going to be asked the "age" question—he was 73—and he prepared with a witty response, probably the most remembered phrase spoken at the debate.

I am not recommending that you tell jokes at your interview; remember, fun is better than funny. The goal is not comedy, but connection. Find the form of humor that works for you and be natural.

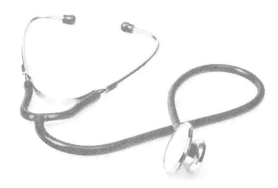

CHAPTER 9

Before the Interview

Okay, now that you are pumped up thinking about how much you're going to learn in this chapter, it's time to go to work! I'm going to break this section down into five easy-to-manage segments:

1. General Preparation
2. Types of Interviews
3. Do's and Don'ts for the PA School Interview
4. Dealing with Anxiety
5. Silencing the "Inner Critic"
6. Final Preparation

Let's get started!

General Preparation

You've done all the work necessary to get your CASPA application completed and submitted. You wait in anticipation to hear back from the PA programs you applied to. One day, you open your email and see that your top choice PA program has sent you a response. You hold your breath, your heart starts pounding, and you quickly open the email. You read, "Congratulations, we would like to extend you an offer to come interview at our PA program." After you jump up and down, call your friends, and soak up the moment, it's now time to prepare for the final, and most difficult, piece of the PA school application process.

You should be very proud of yourself for making it this far, but your job has just begun.

You look great on paper, but you need to show the admissions committee that you look the part in person, too. That means you must begin preparing for your interview long before you stand tall before your interviewer.

The sooner you complete the work, the sooner you can start reviewing the example questions and answers and preparing your own responses. Don't procrastinate; get it done ASAP!

Sleep Hygiene

If you are used to keeping erratic hours, going out with your friends until the early hours of the morning, or just not getting the recommended eight hours of sleep per night, now is the time to get on a regular sleep schedule. You must be fresh every day and have the energy to do the upcoming work necessary to give the performance of your life on the day of your interview.

Take Care of Yourself

If you don't already exercise, start slowly with an exercise routine that will energize you daily. What is the best exercise? The one you'll do! Cut back on your caffeine use. At this point, you should be on a natural "high" anyway. Start eating a healthy diet, low in sugar and high in protein. Get your body running like a well-oiled machine, and by the time your interview comes, you'll be happy, healthy, and confident.

The night before the interview, be sure to arrive to your hotel early (if you're traveling). I strongly recommend that you do a "dry run," and either walk, or drive, to the exact location of the building and room where you will be interviewing the next day. Check out the traffic conditions and the length of time it will take you to get there. Anticipate the worst-case scenario, and leave early in the morning.

You can always go to a restaurant for a small breakfast if you have a lot of spare time. Don't forget to carry the phone number of the program, just in case you hit a traffic jam, or you are going to be late for some other unforeseen reason.

Be sure to eat well the night before your interview. Have a light dinner, and don't eat anything that may linger on your breath. Absolutely no alcohol that night. You certainly don't want to smell like you just came from the bar before your interview.

Take out your suit (yes, wear a suit!), shirt, belt, socks, and shoes. Try everything on BEFORE the interview. Make sure everything looks impeccable: shoes shined, no stains on your clothes, and place everything in a space where you don't have to go searching for items in the morning. You will be nervous enough and you don't need to be frantically searching for your belt for fifteen minutes on the morning of your interview.

Next, take fifteen to twenty minutes to sit quietly in your room. Close your eyes, and visualize your entire interview. See yourself impeccably dressed, confident, answering all the interview questions with ease. This technique is powerful, and it's used by many professional athletes before a big game. A basketball player may visualize herself making every shot she takes, stealing the ball on defense, and grabbing rebound after rebound. This is the equivalent of doing a dry run in your mind.

I always advise bringing a small mirror with you to the interview. You may want to take a close look at your face, teeth, hair, etc. before your interview. Sometimes PA programs offer food and drinks during the day. Having mustard on your face or a piece of broccoli caught between your teeth will certainly not score you any points. And believe me, I've seen it all.

The Day of the Interview

Set your alarm clock to go off early and ask the hotel front desk to provide you with a wake-up call as a back-up. Have a small breakfast before getting dressed. Take a good look in the mirror, and keep your jacket on a hanger while traveling to the interview. Be sure to check yourself again in the bathroom mirror once you're ready to go. Do not overdo the perfume or cologne, and please, no nose rings, tongue rings, or bright pink hair. Now is *not* the time to express yourself in that manner.

I recommend that you arrive at least fifteen minutes early, no sooner, no later. If you are very early, sit in the car or a restaurant, and practice your answers to the questions I have prepared you for. Some applicants like to meditate to calm the nerves. Others like to make a call to some of their friends or a significant other to get some extra support.

Do not bring a cell phone into your interview. You will be too tempted to check text messages, or perhaps sneak in a phone call. Even worse, you don't want your cell phone to ring in the middle of your interview.

Be sure to greet everyone at the program as if they are evaluating you and have a say in the outcome of your interview. If you say the wrong thing to the receptionists, they are likely to pass on this negative experience to one of the committee members that they work with every day, and that will not help your chances. Be friendly and smile at everyone.

Types of Interviews

Many of you will have no idea what to expect when showing up for your PA school interview. I'm not just talking about the questions and answers; I'm talking about the various types of interview formats that you may encounter during this critical phase of the application process. Each program utilizes a format to assess you that will differ depending on what values and qualities they look for in the applicant. You must prepare for each of these formats to give a peak performance. Let's look at the most common formats that you may encounter.

The Solo Interview

The one-on-one interview is the traditional interview format. Your solo interview is typically conducted by a high-level program faculty member. This member is going to have a critical role in the decision-making process, so it goes without saying how crucial this stage is. This solo interviewer will have a key set of qualities and traits that she is looking for, and this is your chance to show her how perfectly you match what she is looking for. Once you finish reading this book, you will feel very comfortable in this traditional interview format. Before you know it, you'll be trying to see where your seat is in the classroom. The best way to do this is to follow the steps I've laid out for you in this book with perfectly tailored answers.

The Panel Interview

Imagine walking through the door and there are three smiling faces staring back at you (or maybe not smiling). This interview format is certainly a bit more anxiety-provoking, but not to worry. There are several reasons why a program uses the panel interview format, but the main reason is to eliminate any bias that one interviewer may have towards an applicant. It also ramps up the pressure a little bit on the applicant, allowing the interviewers to see how well you handle pressure and deal with authority.

To relieve some of the pressure, try to find out beforehand if a panel interview is on the agenda, how many people will be on the panel, and their names, if possible. If the program provides the names of the interviewers, be sure to do some research and find out information about each member. Perhaps one of them won a specific award, or was past president of the American Academy of Physician Assistants (AAPA). Maybe you went to the same college as one of the members, or you both played the same sport. Also, be prepared for the panel to change members on you. Perhaps the three people you've researched conducted an interview with the first applicant of the day, but the panel switches out with three other members for your panel interview. Don't panic! If you've read this book and prepared your own answers to the most common questions, you'll be fine.

One suggestion I have—no, one strong recommendation—is to make eye contact with each member on the panel. For instance, if the interviewer on the left asks you a question, begin answering the question by making eye contact with her for five seconds, then adjusting your gaze to the middle interviewer for five seconds, and next to the interviewer on the right for five seconds. Repeat this process until you've fully answered the question. It is very important to engage everyone at the table, or you risk alienating one of the committee members who may develop a subconscious resentment toward you.

One applicant told me that she was in a panel interview, and one of the interviewers got up in the middle of the session, took a seat behind her, and started asking her questions from a position behind her back. Perhaps this is a technique to see how you handle stress. If this happens to you, remember that eye contact is the key to gaining credibility and trust. So, if this situation happens to you, turn your chair sideways, and look to your left or right so you can establish eye contact with everyone.

The Multiple-Applicant Interview

In my opinion, this is one of the most stressful interviews you will face. You're sitting in a room with other applicants who want *your* seat in the program. Don't worry! I'm going to give you some sure-fire techniques to ensure your voice is heard and you stand out from the crowd in a favorable way. The multiple-applicant interview is a great opportunity to showcase your ability to interact well with others and allows the committee to see if you'd be a good fit for their program. This is a wonderful thing for you if you are using the techniques in this book. Think about it: You'll be in a room full of applicants that aren't using Qualities and Multipliers as part of their responses, and you will certainly stand out from the rest of the applicants.

PA programs love teamwork; it's a trait that is necessary if a class is going to gel and help each other through such an intense program. This type of interview is a great way for the members to see if you play well with others. Are you going to be a team player willing to help others, or a loner who can't be bothered by students who may be having difficulties?

This group interview is not a time to be passive or shy. You want to be assertive, but not aggressive. The interview should create a win-win situation. This is a time to be balanced in your approach. You don't want to be the person who says nothing, and appears to be intimated by the other applicants. On the other hand, you don't want to be the aggressive, chatty know-it-all who thinks he will score high by dominating the other applicants and not allowing them the time to speak. If you want to ace the multiple applicant interview, show your leadership skills by knowing when to speak and when to listen. If someone gives an answer to a question, perhaps you can interject by saying, "I think Sally makes a good point, and I might add..." Do not use the word, "but," because it really means you don't agree with Sally.

The Multiple Mini Interview (MMI)

A multiple mini interview consists of a series of short, structured interview stations used to assess noncognitive qualities, including cultural sensitivity, maturity, teamwork, empathy, reliability, and communication skills.

Prior to the start of each mini-interview rotation, candidates receive a question/scenario and have a designated period to prepare an answer.

Upon entering the interview room, the candidate has a short exchange with an interviewer/assessor. In some situations, the interviewer observes while the action takes place between the applicant and an actor.

At the end of each mini interview, the interviewer evaluates the candidate's performance while the applicant moves to the next station. This pattern is repeated through several rotations. The questions asked are usually situational questions that touch on the following:

- ▸ Ethical decision-making
- ▸ Critical thinking
- ▸ Communication skills
- ▸ Current health care and societal issues

Although participants must relate to the scenario posed at each station, it is important to note that the MMI is not intended to test specific knowledge in the field. Instead, the interviewers evaluate each candidate's thought process and ability to think on their feet. As such, there are no right or wrong answers to the question posed in an MMI, but each applicant should look at the question from a variety of perspectives.

The Student Interview

The student interview usually consists of two or three first- or second-year students asking you questions in a more relaxed format. But don't be fooled by the conversational nature of this interview. The students will have a say on whether they like you or not, particularly evaluating you as someone they would like to have as a classmate. Treat the students with the utmost respect. Look at this interview as a fantastic opportunity to let them sell you on why you should attend their program.

You're not likely to be asked traditional interview questions in the student interview, but if you've followed the guidance in this book, you'll be prepared to discuss Qualities and Multipliers that you've researched before the interview. Be sure to visit the student society website or blog to find out what unique events or projects students are involved in. Students are very proud of their program and the events they participate in. Perhaps a group of students went on a mission trip to South America to provide vaccinations to children in isolated regions of a country. It would be nice to know this information ahead of time. Take the time to do your homework and let the students know that you have the same values and Qualities as they have.

Do's and Don'ts for the PA School Interview

Now that you know how to prepare for the various PA school interviews you may encounter, let's take a list of DOs and DON'Ts.

Do...

Do your homework (research)! Learn everything you can about the program(s) where you will be interviewing. Start early. The program's website is the first place to start. Leave no stone unturned. View every page and link on the site. Don't forget about social media, either. Check out the program on Facebook, Google, blogs, student sites, and YouTube. For example, I found the following about the Barry University PA Program using Google:

> **No More Tears Charity Golf Tournament**
> *by Barry University PA Program*
> EVENT DETAILS
>
> A group of motivated, **civic-minded** Barry University Physician Assistant Students have committed to raising money and awareness for the No More Tears Project. No More Tears is a 100% not-for-profit organization that is operated entirely through the **selfless** efforts of volunteers and donors whose **mission is to rescue the victims of domestic violence and human trafficking.**

How many applicants do you think will know about this event on interview day? Can you infuse these Qualities and the Multiplier in some of the answers to interview questions at Barry? The Qualities are listed, and the Multiplier is the event.

DON'T... Continuously call the program and become a nuisance. Don't ask questions that you should know from searching the program's website.

DO... Invest in a suit if you don't have one. You may be able to rent a suit, also. The point is, always lean toward overdressing rather than underdressing.

DON'T... Come to the interview with nose rings, tongue rings, flashy jewelry, low-cut blouses, unkempt hair, or a wrinkled outfit. Dress for success. You want the focus to be on you, not your attire.

DO... Eat a simple, well-balanced meal the night before your interview—and a good breakfast the morning of.

DON'T... Eat a bunch of spicy food, or junk food, the night before your interview. You don't want to have acid reflux first thing in the morning, which will make you feel miserable. Do not drink alcohol before your interview to calm your nerves. I will teach you a much better way to deal with anxiety later in the book.

DO... Get a good night's sleep the night before your interview.

DON'T... Stay up all night stressing over the interview, or cramming information into your brain. Reassure yourself that you are prepared, watch a movie, and relax as best you can.

DO... Take a shower, brush your teeth, and spend the time to look your best. As you already know, the visual component of an interview will weigh significantly on your score.

DON'T... Smoke before your interview; your clothes will smell of tobacco and being a smoker is not the best way to show that you are an advocate for health.

DO... Arrive early to your interview, review your notes, and practice the anxiety relieving technique that I will teach you later.

DON'T... be rude to *anyone* you meet at the program, including the other applicants. For example, if the receptionist asks you, "Did you have any trouble finding us?" your response should be, "Absolutely not! You gave excellent directions, thank you." You'll want to start things off on a positive note.

DO... Be a real person. In other words, do your best to be likeable, trustworthy, and credible.

DON'T... Panic. Remember, it's not about *you*, it's about them. Get out of your own head and shut off that inner critic. You are prepared for this interview. Remember that the committee wants you to solve their problem—finding the perfect applicant who has all the Qualities *they* are looking for.

Dealing with Anxiety

Here is a technique to quiet your mind and relieve the anxiety that you are likely to feel on the day of your interview.

As soon as you open your eyes on the morning of your interview, I can assure you that your heart will start racing, your breath will be shallow and rapid, and you will probably have a knot in the pit of your stomach. Don't panic! What you're experiencing is healthy anxiety. Your body's physiology is acting appropriately. The challenge is to avoid panicking.

As an example, think about the following situation: You come out of your friend's house and begin walking to your car. You suddenly hear loud barking, and a huge dog, foaming at the mouth, is making a beeline right toward you. Your physiology begins to go into fight-or-flight mode; your pupils immediately dilate, your breathing becomes rapid and shallow, and your heart rate goes through the roof. I think it's safe to say that at a time like this, it's not exactly the best moment to do your taxes. So, if you want to be able to think clearly, particularly on the day of your interview, you need to control your physiology because you're likely to be in fight-or-flight mode when you enter the building.

If you are not prepared for this on the day of your interview, your plan is to "wing it." This plan is going to cause a lot more anxiety, and you will be in the fight-or-flight mode throughout the entire interview process. You will have a very difficult time answering interview questions if you can't change this physiological response.

Dr. Eva Selhub, a mind/body expert, resiliency coach, motivational speaker, and executive coach, teaches a powerful technique used to instantly reduce a person's stress and anxiety level. Her technique is to put up your SHIELD™. You can use this technique while waiting to be called into the room, and nobody will have to know that you're using it. The SHIELD™ acronym stands for:

Stop
Honor the feeling
Inhale
Exhale
Listen
Decide

Author of *The Love Response*, Dr. Selhub promotes a simple philosophy: At its best, stress motivates. At its worst, stress annihilates. Good leaders motivate. Bad leaders annihilate.

The choice is yours to decide how stress will influence your leadership. If you find yourself in an anxiety-provoking or stressful situation (like the PA school interview), you can use the SHIELD™ technique to instantly change your physiology.

If you utilize this technique, your breathing will slow down, your heart rate will decrease, your pupils will return to normal size, and you will be able to think much more clearly.

Here is how the technique works:

▸ Once you feel your anxiety level becoming too high, *stop* what you are doing.

▸ Then, *honor the feeling* (non-judgmentally). Are you anxious, afraid, frustrated, angry, lonely, or tired?

▸ Next, *inhale and exhale*, ten times in a row. (When you breathe in, imagine filling an empty balloon in your belly with your breath. When you breathe out, imagine deflating the balloon.) Repeat the breaths ten times, and you will notice a soothing, calming effect. By this time, your adrenaline is dropping, and you will be able to think clearly and focus on the task at hand.

- Now, *listen* to your mind and become aware of your thoughts and feelings and *decide* to ace your interview.
- You've worked hard, you're prepared, and you deserve a seat in the class.

You can repeat the above technique as many times as necessary to help you relax and focus.

Silencing the Inner Critic

In a variety of stressful situations, we become our own worst enemy. I can remember arriving for my interview at Yale and meeting my competition. Everyone in the room had a master's degree, except for me. My inner critic came alive. "I'm never going to get in!" I was being very hard on myself and extremely judgmental. Negative self-talk only serves to perpetuate the anxiety and make things worse.

Here are some things *your* inner critic may shout at you on the day of your interview:

- "I should have prepared more."
- "Everyone here is more qualified than I am."
- "I'll never get accepted."
- "I'm a loser; I don't belong here."
- "I'm going to blow this interview."

Don't wait until your interview to address your inner critic. Here are some steps that you can take to deal with your inner critic weeks or months before your interview:

1. **Monitor your thoughts.** Becoming aware of your inner critic's voice—if you will—is the first step. You can achieve this by simply being mindful of those thoughts. Just notice when and where the thoughts occur, and then write them down on a piece

of paper or in a journal. You may become acutely aware of certain patterns in your thinking. Once you master being mindful and get the negative thoughts on paper, you can begin to silence the inner critic.

2. **Notice your judgments.** Instead of making judgments, try describing your thoughts or feelings. For example, you may be having a conversation with a fellow student about a class you are both taking. You may really like the professor, and during the conversation, you might say, "Professor Jones is a great teacher." Your classmate might not agree with you and say, "I think he's a terrible teacher." Both of you are making judgments and possibly putting the other person on guard to defend his or her decision.

   If you said instead, "I appreciate that Professor Jones always comes prepared to class. It makes it easier for me to stay focused." You are not being judgmental; you are simply describing the way you *feel* about him. Nobody can dispute that, not even your friend. The point is that when we are being judgmental, especially of ourselves, we promote more intense feelings of negativity. And at the interview, we want to stay positive.

3. **Challenge your automatic negative thoughts.** Feelings aren't facts! Once you practice mindfulness and become good at documenting your thoughts (judgments), it is time to challenge those negative thoughts with the facts. You may feel like you don't have what it takes to be accepted, but if you look at the facts, you may change your mind.

   For example, if you were to review your CASPA application, you would see that you've worked hard to complete the requirements for PA school. The fact that you received an offer to interview means that you've already beat out several hundred applicants to get the interview. So, although you may certainly feel like you don't have what it takes to get accepted, the facts prove otherwise. Try to challenge all your negative thoughts with the facts. Chances are, you will find that you are beating yourself up for no reason.

4. **Practice, not perfection.** The goal of practicing mindfulness and keeping your judgments in check is to achieve awareness and make gradual changes. Becoming aware of the problem is the first step. However, if you are in denial about how your judgments and negative thoughts affect your mindset, you will not be able to make any progress at all. It takes constant vigilance to achieve improvement with mindfulness.

5. **Reconsider your values.** Make sure that whatever you are beating yourself up over is worth striving for. Some goals, like kindness, integrity, and being self-disciplined, enhance the meaning and quality of life, whereas others only feed into your sense of defectiveness. Some people think, *If I only went to a better school, I'd have more self-esteem.* By the way, the best way to increase self-esteem is to do esteemable things!

Final Preparation

Remember, your job at the interview is to help make the interviewer's job easy by showing her that you have the qualities and values she is looking for in a perfect applicant. It's not about you, it's about them. Your interviewer is not out to trip you up. She's a regular person, with a family, worries, and insecurities just like you. In fact, she may be as nervous as you are.

Be prepared for multiple interviews. I recommend that you call the program beforehand to see if they will tell you how many interviews you will have, and perhaps even who will be your interviewers. Find out if they use traditional questions, behavioral questions, or a multiple mini interview (MMI) format.

From the time you enter the building until the time you exit, you are being evaluated. Maintain a professional appearance and attitude throughout the entire process. Greet everyone with a smile and a handshake, from the Dean of the program to the custodian vacuuming the floors. Remember that, although you may only be there for one day, these people spend forty hours a week together, just like in any other job. They're like a small family, and they've seen a lot of candidates come and go. If you say something negative or controversial in front of the receptionist, don't be surprised if she passes that information on to the committee members. You've done too much work to be here, it would be a tragedy to be rejected because you insulted one of the staff.

Finally, be sure to treat the student interviewers with the utmost respect. Don't let your guard down because you think students don't have much of a say with respect to scoring your interview. Take advantage of the opportunity to ask what they like most about the program, and what Qualities the program values. Your goal should be to convince the students that you've worked hard to be here and that you would make a great classmate. You must be likeable.

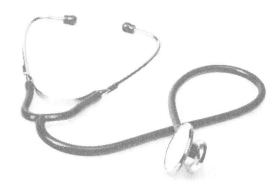

CHAPTER 10

Dressing for Interviews

After following the PA Forum (physicianassistantforum.com) for two decades, I can honestly say that one frequently asked question is, "Should I wear a suit to my interview?"

Maybe it's because I'm old school, but I just don't get this question. The cynical part of me wants to respond, "Well, everyone else will be wearing a suit to this *professional* interview, but *you* can probably wear jeans and pull it off!"

I know that most of you are not considering wearing jeans, but you may want to know if it's okay to wear a sport coat and dress pants, or a grey suit versus a blue suit. Below I'm going to provide you with a complete list of what to wear to your PA school interview.

Remember, there are three components to the spoken message: the verbal component, the vocal component, and the visual component. The visual component counts for fifty-five percent of your message at your interview. When in doubt, dress up!

Men

✓ Remember that you are dressing for a professional interview and what you wear needs to be appropriate for the occasion. This means wearing a suit! It is not appropriate to dress down for your PA school interview, unless you want to give a negative impression as soon as you walk through the door. When in doubt, dress conservatively.

✓ Wearing a "suit" means the whole package: a matching jacket and pants, dress shirt (preferably white), a tie, coordinating socks and dress shoes (shined). A dark-colored suit with a light-colored tie is your best option.

✓ You suit should be comfortable and fit you well so that you look and act your best. If your ten-year-old suit doesn't fit well, invest in a new one.

✓ Avoid loud colors and flashy ties.

✓ Your clothing should be neat, clean, and freshly pressed. I recommend you keep your suit, tie, and shirt in the dry-cleaning package until the morning of your interview. Be sure to shower, shave, and wear deodorant the morning of your interview. Do not wear cologne or aftershave, and certainly do not smoke before your interview.

✓ Make sure you have fresh breath. Brush your teeth before your interview, and don't eat before the interview.

✓ Your hair should be neat, clean, and conservative.

✓ Shoes should be well-polished, in good condition, and the appropriate color to match your suit.

✓ Be sure to shave before the interview. If you have a mustache or beard, it should be trimmed and neat.

Women

✓ Wear a suit. Either a skirt or pants is fine.

✓ Your suit should be comfortable and fit well.

✓ Your suit should be simple and dark in color. Anything tight, bright, short, or sheer should absolutely be avoided. Interviewers notice everything, and if your skirt is too short it could work against you. If you have any doubts about the length of your skirt, it's probably too short. Knee-length skirts are recommended. Maxi skirts are also considered too trendy for an interview.

✓ Wear a conservative blouse with your suit. Do not wear bright colors, animal prints, or anything lacy, sheer, or low-cut.

✓ Makeup and nail polish should be understated and flattering; shades that are neutral to your skin tone are generally advisable. Avoid bright or unusual colors or very long nails.

✓ Keep jewelry and hair accessories to a minimum, and stick to those that are not flashy, distracting, or shiny. Only one ring per hand.

✓ Shoes should be conservative and low-healed. They should be in good shape, and well shined. Don't wear shoes with an open toe or back; any shoes that you would wear on a date or to a club are probably inappropriate. A basic pump is flattering, versatile, and will stay in style forever.

✓ If you intend to wear them, your hose should be neutral (matched to your skin tone). Carry an extra pair of hose in case you rip the ones you have on.

✓ Your clothes should be neat, clean, and freshly pressed.

✓ Shower on the morning of your interview. Wear deodorant, but no perfume in case your interviewer has an allergy.

✓ Brush your teeth in the morning, and don't eat, drink, or smoke afterward.

✓ Your hair should be neat, clean, and conservatively styled. Banana clips, bright-colored scrunchies or elastics, and cheerleader-type ponytails look out of place with a suit. You may consider wearing an updo, pulling it back into a low ponytail, or wearing a simple barrette. The idea is to look polished and professional, not to advertise what a creative genius your hairdresser is.

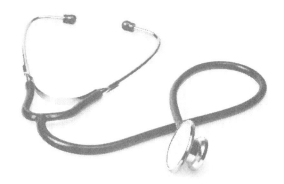

CHAPTER 11

Frequently Asked Questions (FAQs)

Q: How do I answer questions about Fs or Ws on my transcripts?
A: I always tell applicants to live by three rules at your interview: Be honest, be yourself, and accept responsibility. I recommend that you reread your CASPA application a few days before your interview and look for any potential deficiencies that you may need to address, with poor grades being one of them.

Whatever the reason for the Fs or Ws, take responsibility and *don't make excuses*. Realize that you wouldn't be at an interview if those grades were going to be disqualifiers. The committee just wants to understand why you've done well in your other classes, but not these.

Q: Should I take notes during my interview?

A: I recommend that you bring a pad and pen to your interview. Typically, before you get into the interview process, you will have a briefing or two from the Dean of the program, or even from the financial aid officer. It is perfectly fine to take notes during this time. I *do not recommend taking notes* during your interview for two reasons:

1. Many programs do not allow you to take notes during the interview, out of concern for applicants writing down the interview questions, and perhaps sharing them with others.
2. If you are taking notes, you can't maintain eye contact with the interviewers. That would be a fatal mistake.

Q: Should I ask questions during the tour of the school?

A: Absolutely! In many cases, the tour guide is asked to report back to the admissions committee on those applicants who stood out, for good reasons or bad. This is the perfect time to ask a lot of questions about the Qualities the school values. Knowing the Qualities will make it much easier for you to infuse them into your interview answers.

If the tour is after your interview, you want to be on your best behavior and ask questions that are relevant to the program. Again, a negative report back to the committee could ruin your chances of acceptance.

Q: What are *underserved* populations?

A: Medically underserved areas/populations are areas of populations designated by the Health Resources and Services Administration (HRSA) as having too few primary care providers, high infant mortality, high poverty, or high elderly populations.

Q: Should I mention the specialty area where I want to practice after graduating?

A: I highly recommend you don't do this. As a former admissions committee member, whenever an applicant mentions the word "specialty," I feel that they are close-minded. How does the applicant already know what area of medicine they would like to practice if they've never worked in that area as a PA? Many applicants may want to work in the Emergency Room because they had an enjoyable experience as an ER tech. However, being a tech in the ER and being a PA in the ER are two different experiences.

I personally loved being an ER tech and *knew* I wanted to work in the ER once I graduated. However, after doing a clinical rotation in the ER as a PA student, I realized being a clinician in the ER was not for me. After doing all my rotations, I found that Cardiac Surgery was where I wanted to work.

But what about primary care, you may be asking? Don't most programs want their students to work in primary care? Many PA school websites state that their mission is to produce graduates to work in primary care or in underserved areas. In reality, most graduates do not take jobs in primary care.

Personally, based on my twenty-four years to date, working as a PA in five different areas of medicine, is that I wish I started my career in family practice. I currently work in family practice, and I found myself way behind the eight-ball when I joined the group four years ago. I always worked in specialty areas of medicine, and I never built the solid foundation that a family practice position offers. Coming out of school and working in family practice is a terrific way to add to your fund of knowledge from PA school, as well as reinforce that knowledge with clinical experience. A solid foundation will serve you well no matter where you might end up working.

Q: What if I'm asked questions about my political opinions?

A: Run for your life! This country is in political turmoil right now. Everyone has strong opinions, whether you're a Democrat, Republican, or Independent. You have no idea what the political views of your interviewer(s) are. If your interviewer is a staunch Democrat and you let her know that you are a Republican, she may, unknowingly, automatically develop a bias toward you. I advise you to come right out and say, "It is my policy to never discuss politics with friends, and certainly not in an interview."

Q: Is it okay to bring my parents to the interview?

A: It is okay for your parents to travel with you to the interview city/town for support, but you should not bring them to the actual interview. One of the qualities admissions committees look for is maturity. Bringing your parents with you to the interview may be taken as a sign of immaturity.

Q: Do you have any tips on the group interview?

A: First off, be sure you understand what the program means by "group" interview. It could mean that you will meet with a group of interviewers (usually three) and are the only candidate. Or, it can mean that you and a group of other students will meet in a round table type discussion. I'll assume for this question that we're talking about the latter.

In group interviews, you will be in a room with several other applicants and perhaps one or two interviewers. The interviewer will ask each of you the same question and go around the table until each applicant has had the opportunity to answer the question.

Many times, in the group interview session, applicants will simply parrot what the first applicant says, even if she didn't fully answer the question. That appears to be the effortless way out. You are not going to stand out from the other applicants if you do so.

I recommend that when it's your turn to answer the question, ask the interviewer to repeat the question, or you repeat it back to him and ask, "Do I have that right?" This way you will know exactly what the interviewer is asking, and you will be sure you're answering the question being asked.

If one of the applicants answers the question well, I recommend that you say, "I agree with Susan about..., and I think I would add..." This is your opportunity to bring something to the table. You will have to focus and think on your feet. Be sure not to say, "I agree with Susan, *but*..." Saying "but" really means you don't agree with Susan. Using "and" is a much better way to phrase it.

Tips for the group interview:

- ▸ Be sure to make eye contact with everyone in the room when answering a question. You want to show the committee that you are inclusive, even with your competition.

► Be sure to smile during this interview.

► Don't be a know-it-all. Some applicants think the more they talk, the better the impression they'll make with the committee. Nothing could be further from the truth. If you dominate the conversation, it may show that you are not a team player, and you are not respecting your potential future classmates. This interview is not a contest; it's a way for the interviewers to get to know you and see if you would be a good fit for their program.

► Be sure to answer the question!

► If the committee throws out a question for anyone to answer, raise your hand. It's the polite thing to do, and you won't have to talk over everyone else. You'll get your chance to answer, and the committee will appreciate you giving everyone an equal chance. It's not about how many questions you answer, but the quality of your answers—and by now you are an expert at infusing Qualities into your answers.

Q: Should I bring my purse to the interview?

A: I would recommend keeping your purse locked up in your car. I can see no reason why you would need it at your interview. Even if they ask you to bring a driver's license or any other documents, place them in a folder and hand them to the receptionist. If you feel a burning desire to bring your purse with you, leave it in the orientation room and do not bring it into the interview room.

Also, *do not* bring your cell phone under any circumstances!

Q: Should I bring my resume to the interview?

A: Do not bring a resume unless asked to do so. They have your CASPA application, which contains everything they need to know about you. The committee reviews thousands of documents to select candidates; believe me, they don't want to have to read another one. You made it to the interview, and your resume won't add to your application. In fact, when I was on the admissions committee, we ruled a woman out because of totally inappropriate things she included in her resume.

Q: What if the answer to a question is on the tip of my tongue, but I can't recall it at the exact time they ask me?

A: It is very human for all of us to forget someone's name, or an answer to a test question. Many times, the answer is right on the tip of our tongue, but it just won't come exactly at the time we need it. If this happens to you, don't try to ramble and fill in the time with an unintelligible answer. That will not help you. Instead, be honest! Tell the committee that the answer is right on the tip of your tongue, but you can't recall it right now. Ask if it's okay to proceed to the next question, to buy some time and allow your subconscious brain to come up with the answer for you.

As an example, have you ever noticed an old classmate walking toward you and you panic because you cannot remember her name? This has happened to all of us. It can be awkward, and we are usually hoping the name will pop into our head right at that moment. But, when does the name come to you? Typically, as soon as you walk away! Your subconscious was working on finding her name the whole time, but it usually takes a few minutes to retrieve the information. The admissions committee will appreciate your honesty, rather than listen to you make up a response and embarrass yourself.

Q: Can I use humor during my interview?

A: Humor can be a powerful way to loosen up the interviewer(s), but if it backfires it can ruin the interview. There are times when humor can be used effectively, though. If you are asked, "Which ninja turtle would you be?" You can jokingly say, with a smile on your face, "I was just thinking about that last night." Humor is okay, but telling jokes in not a promising idea.

Q: Should I send "thank you" letters?

A: I often get asked this question after my coaching applicants return home from their interview. There are two schools of thought on this topic. One is that the admissions committee has probably scored your application by the time you leave the interview. At this point, sending a thank you letter is not going to help your score. Personally, I never received a thank you letter while I was on the ADCOM at Yale, and it didn't bother me. Again, just one more paper to read.

The other school of thought is that it can't hurt, and it's polite. However, don't expect that a thank you letter will increase your score.

Q: Do I have to wear a suit?

A: This question always makes me smile. Sometimes my sarcastic response is, "No, you don't have to wear a suit. Everyone else will be wearing one, but you can probably pull it off wearing jeans." I know, very sarcastic, and I don't mean to offend anyone. But, yes—wear a suit! End of story.

Q: What if I get interview offers from two schools for the same day?

A: Being asked to interview on the same day at two different schools is not as uncommon as you may think. If this happens to you, first congratulate yourself on getting two interviews! Clearly you are a strong applicant.

Then, decide which of the two schools you would choose to attend if selected to both. Once you figure that out, call the other program and tell them that you have a scheduling conflict for the day of your interview, and would they mind providing you with another date.

This scenario is very common, and most programs are flexible when it comes to rescheduling.

Q: Can you suggest any books that I can read if they ask me about this?

A: Yes, I found these recommendations on the PA Forum (physician-assistantforum.com):

- ▸ *Night,* by Elie Wiesel
- ▸ *Moloka'i,* by Alan Brennert
- ▸ *The Book Thief,* by Markus Zusak

Q: Are new programs easier to get accepted to than more established programs?

A: This is certainly a legitimate question. Many applicants feel that they will have a better chance for acceptance if the program is brand new. I have a different opinion on this answer, but let's look at some of the pros and cons of going to a brand-new program:

▶ **Pros**

You will have the opportunity to be an inaugural class member. The faculty will be fresh and will be committed to helping their program succeed.

Most new programs rely on more established PA programs to help them set up a curriculum. The new program will bring in a lot of wisdom from other programs with a proven track record.

Many times, the faculty of a new program are experienced faculty members from previous programs; they will bring their experience to the new program as well.

▶ **Cons**

In my experience, first year programs typically have a lot more applicants than established programs. I believe applicants think a newer program is easier to get into, because less people apply than an established program. I believe the opposite is true.

One of the top priorities of a newer program is to establish high PANCE rates on the boards. If a new program's PANCE rates are below the national average (94%), applicants may eventually start shying away from applying to that program. They may feel they are not going to be prepared very well for the boards, and it would be risky to take the chance on this new program.

My biggest concern with new PA programs relates to their clinical rotation sites. It can take several years for an established PA program to find an excellent clinical experience in each of the specialty areas for their students.

At Yale, we had a folder on every clinical rotation site that the students could read through when selecting where they wanted to do each rotation. Inside that folder were critiques from former students. Perhaps one of the students noted, "The medical students had top priority on this rotation. Medical students were assigned all the challenging cases, and the PAs were on the bottom of the totem pole," or "The supervising physician seemed too busy to provide a lot of teaching. I felt that I did not learn as much as I wanted. Very disappointing."

Why are clinical rotations so important? From my own experience, I found that what I learned on clinical rotations significantly helped me answer many board questions on the PANCE. I would remember the clinical experience more than I would remember learning about it in the classroom.

If you don't have established clinical rotation sites, your preceptors may not be the best teachers, or you may not learn as much as you should because they cater to the medical students over the PA students. It could take several years for a program to establish excellent rotation sites.

A new PA program may start with provisional accreditation. If they don't achieve full accreditation by the time you graduate, you won't be able to sit for the boards.

Q: Should I mention a DUI or DWI that I have on my record?

A: My mantra for applying to PA school and for the PA school interview is to be honest and be real. The CASPA application requires applicants to identify any arrests, misdemeanors included. You need to mention the DUI/DWI. What I recommend you do, however, is to dedicate a small paragraph in your essay to explain the circumstances and what you've learned from the experience.

Clearly a DUI/DWI will be viewed as irresponsible and demonstrating poor judgment. I would not leave the reader of your application wondering what the circumstances were. Give a brief explanation in your essay and be prepared to discuss the offense at your interview. Do not make excuses!

Q: I have a Bad Conduct Discharge from the Air Force. Can I still get into PA school?

A: I've come across this situation many times when coaching PA school applicants. You must disclose this information. The best route to go is to try and get the Bad Conduct Discharge (BCD) expunged.

If you are unable to get the BCD expunged, you should set up a meeting with the Dean of the program(s) you are applying to and try to get some feedback as to how they will view the BCD. Some programs may not be as concerned as others. It will also likely depend on why you received a BCD. If your BCD resulted from an assault or sexual harassment, you're likely not going to be accepted. If the BCD resulted from having a urine with marijuana in it, you may have a better chance.

Don't try to sweep this issue under the carpet. Approach it head-on and hope for the best.

Q: I applied last year, and I was not accepted to any of the programs I applied to; will that hurt my application this year?

A: PA school is extremely competitive, and it's certainly a numbers game. The fact is, most applicants do not get accepted any given year. It doesn't mean you're a bad applicant, it just means there are a lot of good applicants.

The only way you can hurt yourself for the next cycle is if you do nothing to improve your application. Before reapplying, take more classes, get more medical experience, and shadow more PAs. You may be asked the question in the interview, "So, what have you done to strengthen your application this year?"

I've covered some of the most frequent questions I am asked from my applicants who participate in mock interviews with me. There will always be more questions.

Feel free to email me at **andyrodican@gmail.com** if you have any questions not covered in the FAQs. For further information or to schedule a mock interview, visit my website at **andrewrodican.com**.

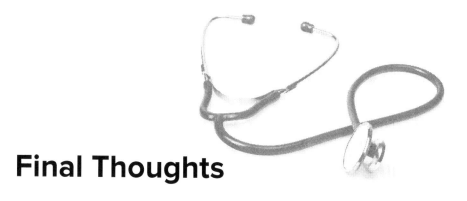

Final Thoughts

I hope by now you're feeling much more confident preparing for your upcoming PA school interview. I can promise you that by reading this book, you will be exponentially more prepared than applicants who have not.

You now have a blueprint for answering any type of interview questions. You do not have to memorize answers; instead, just follow the blueprint and practice the questions prior to your interview. Think more in terms of Qualities, and how you can demonstrate them to the committee. Always remember, *it's not about you, it's about them*. Your goal is to become the *Perfect* Applicant, not a *vanilla* applicant. By infusing Qualities into your answers, you are telling the committee that you have exactly what they're looking for, and a great fit for the program.

Practice the SHIELD™ technique to reduce your anxiety. It is perfectly normal to be anxious on the day of your interview, but you do not want to become paralyzed because your adrenaline is sky-high, and you are in fight-or-flight mode. The SHIELD™ technique works on your body's physiology and is guaranteed to lower adrenaline levels.

Reread the chapter, "Winning through High Impact Communication." Remember the visual component of the interview is the most valuable component. Make eye contact, use open gestures, and smile.

Additionally, avoid speaking in a monotone. Put your voice on a roller coaster and speak with passion. Show that you are extremely motivated to be there and to become a PA school student.

Finally, don't forget to prepare as much as you can for your interview(s.) *Failure to prepare, is preparing to fail.* If you think you can go into your interview and "wing it," you're in for a rude awakening. Read this book, incorporate the ideas from this book, and do a mock interview. It doesn't have to be with me, but make sure you do it with someone who has experience with the PA school interview process and has experience with multiple programs in the country. Many PAs are willing to give you advice; just remember their experience is usually from the program they attended. I've been doing this for over twenty years and have worked with applicants from almost every program in the country.

Most applicants realize after doing a mock interview, how unprepared they really are. Reading about the interview process is the polar opposite of answering interview questions live. I have hundreds of testimonials from applicants who were accepted to PA school, thanking me for preparing them during their mock interview.

The investment for the mock interview is negligible relative to the investment you will make paying for PA school. You will probably spend more money on your stethoscope than a mock interview.

I wish you the best of luck on your journey to become a PA. Whether you will become a physician assistant or a physician associate, you are about to enter one of the best career fields in the country. I have never regretted one day of my twenty-four-year career.

Perhaps we'll meet one day in the future as colleagues!

ABOUT THE AUTHOR

Andrew J. Rodican, PA-C, is a 1994 graduate of the Yale University Physician
Associate Program, and a recipient of
the Yale PA Program Medical Writing
Award. Andrew served for three years
on Yale's PA program's admissions
committee, both as a student and an
alumni member. He is currently a Clinical Adjunct Professor at the Quinnipiac
University School of Health Sciences
Physician Assistant Program.

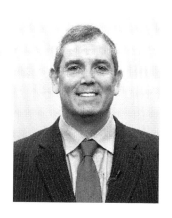

In 1996, Rodican self-published *The Ultimate Guide to Getting Into Physician Assistant School*, the first book ever published for PA school applicants. The book sold so many copies and received so much praise from PA school applicants, that it was published in 1997 by Appleton & Lange, and in 2004 by McGraw-Hill. It is currently in its fourth edition and considered the bible for PA school applicants.

Over the past twenty years, Andrew has traveled the country, giving live seminars to applicants in many states. He has also published three more books for PA school applicants. His website, andrewrodican.com, provides free tips, resources, and coaching, with essay review and edits for PA school applicants.

Andrew has also done hundreds of mock interviews via Skype with applicants from every state in the country, who are applying to almost every PA school in the country. Applicants can sign up for a mock interview or an essay review on Rodican's website.

With over twenty-four years of experience, Andrew Rodican has become a PA school admissions committee expert, and a pioneer in field of PA school coaching.

OTHER BOOKS BY ANDREW RODICAN, PA-C

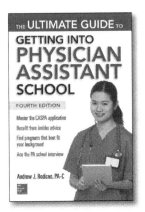

The Ultimate Guide to Getting Into Physician Assistant School, Fourth Edition

304 pages, McGraw-Hill Education, 2017
ISBN 978-1-2598-5984-7
Available on Amazon.com

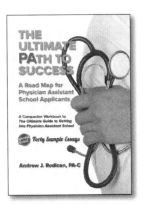

The Ultimate PAth to Success: A Roadmap for Physician Assistant School Applicants

240 pages, Createspace, 2016
ISBN 978-1-5197-0577-8
Available on Amazon.com and andrewrodican.com

VISIT MY WEBSITE
andrewrodican.com

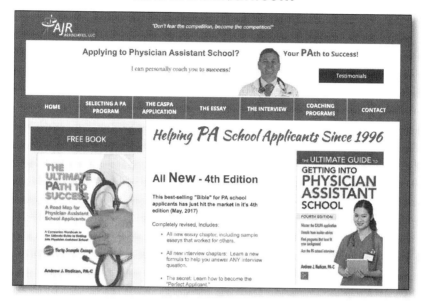

How to Ace the Physician Assistant School Interview is the #1 selling book for Physician Assistant School Applicants on amazon.com. If you read this book and incorporate my Tailoring Method for answering *any* interview question, you will have a significant advantage over your competition. This book will take you from a "vanilla" applicant, to the Perfect Applicant.

Additionally, many applicants will go into their interview and try to "wing it." I offer a Mock Interview service where I will personally conduct a two-hour Skype interview with you. I cover a variety of questions, and help you formulate answers to some of the toughest interview questions you will be asked.

The PA school interview may be the most important interview of your life. Why go it alone? Let my twenty-years of experience help you blow away the competition! Visit my website for more information.

INTERVIEW NOTES

INTERVIEW NOTES

INTERVIEW NOTES

Made in the USA
Columbia, SC
08 December 2021